Unraveling and Re-Birth

*Its name
Is Public Opinion
It is held in reverence.
It settles everything.
Some think it is
The voice of God.
Loyalty to petrified opinion never yet
Broke a chain
Or freed a human soul.*

Mark Twain

*I cannot give you
The formula for success,
But I can give you the formula
For failure which is:
Try to please everybody.*

Herbert Bayard Swope

Acknowledgements

This book is the cumulative effort of three years of travel, interviews, focus groups, literature reviews, and reading survey documents. I'm grateful to Personnel Decisions International, especially Lowell Hellervik, CEO, for the encouragement and support to engage in this healthcare research project.

To the more than five hundred physicians and healthcare leaders and more than a hundred patients who gave of your time, energy, and passion in one-to-one interviews, written response questionnaires, and focus groups, I want you to know that your voice was heard and will hopefully be taken seriously by everyone who has a stake in our healthcare future.

While I would like to list the names of everyone involved in this project, I will honor the promise to maintain anonymity. This book would not have been possible without the candid and unguarded comments and stories provided by all of you. If it were possible I would Knight all of you and nominate you for Sainthood. I can do the latter.

My colleagues at Zobius Leadership International, Bob Terry, Mo Fahnestock, and Rob Kreiger, Ron Hultgren, Judie Ramsey, and Michael LaBrosse have reviewed this book and allowed me to suffer the inaccuracies and take responsibility for them; they act with strong wills, humility and authenticity. The sequel to this book is already being framed and will deal with the paradigm shifts, losses, and learning disabilities.

To my many physician and healthcare executive friends, Mary Jo Lewis, Rodney Dueck, Bruce Pitts, Ron Peterson, Jeevan Paul, Jim Smith, Julie Blehm, Bret Haake, Subbarao Inampudi, Jim Tuscanco, Brian Campion, Bob Olson, Mark Arnesen, Michael Tedford, Marques Rhoades, Tom Gilliam, Warren Green, Wayne Hoffman, John Toso, Bjorn Flygenring, Zachary Gerbarg, Joel Koenig, David Page, Thomas Spence, Michael Trangle, Bill Peterson, Roger Gilbertson, Jamie Peters, David Larson, Wm. Clover, Randall Claw, who read, discussed, and offered valuable insights and additions, I am deeply grateful.

Brian Campion, MD, author of the chapter on partnerships, is a model of strong will and humility, the characteristics essential for effective physician leadership. He leads the Physician Leadership College at the University of St. Thomas. I appreciate his friendship, humor, and guidance.

As for my best friend, Marian, I continue to marvel at her patience, beauty of soul and depth of commitment. I'm fortunate to have such a life partner.

The Unraveling And Re-Birth Of Healthcare

Warren M. Hoffman

A DayBreak Publication

Warren M. Hoffman, Ph.D.
Principle

Zobius Leadership International

**Personal
Professional &
Organizational
Authenticity**

646 Dale Court S.
St. Paul, Minnesota 55126
651-484-3940
warrenhoffman@zobius.net
www.zobius.net

The Unraveling and Re-Birth of Healthcare
Copyright 2002 Warren M. Hoffman

All rights reserved. No part of this book may be reproduced, stores in a retrieval system, or transmitted, in any form or by any means, electronic, mechanical, photocopying, recording, or otherwise, without the prior written permission of the publisher.

Discounts on bulk quantities are available to corporation, professional associations and other organizations. For details contact DayBreak1@attbi.com

Library of Congress Cataloging-in-Publication Data
Healthcare
Library of Congress control number: 2002093991

ISBN: 0-940916-12-6
10 9 8 7 6 5 4 3 2 1

Published by DayBreak
Cover Photography Copyright © 1997 Morris Press
Printed in the United States of America by Morris Publishing
First Edition

Table Of Contents

	Paradigm Shifts in Healthcare	6
	7 Losses of Physicians	7
	Learning Disabilities in Healthcare	7
	Executive Summary	8
Chapter 1ne	Changing Landscape of Healthcare	11
Chapter 2wo	Unraveling Chaos	29
Chapter 3hree	Survey and Responses	51
Chapter 4our	Learning Disabilities in HealthCare	93
Chapter 5ive	Competencies of the Physician Leader	103
Chapter 6ix	Power and Leadership	119
Chapter 7even	Teams and Multi-Disciplinary Decision-Making	139
Chapter 8ight	Partnerships: Brian Campion	155
Chapter 9ine	Polarities and Paradox Re-Visited	161
Chapter 10en	Re-Birth of HealthCare	167
Chapter 11even	Physician leaders introduced	171
Author		176
Bibliography		177

Paradigm Shifts in Healthcare

From	*To*
Primary focus on physician	Focus on patients/partnerships
Teaching medical students	Creating learning environments
Individual focus	Team focus
Discrete disciplines	Inter-disciplinary
Isolated specialties	Integrated practices
Discipline-based practice	Wellness (illness prevention) based practice
Homogenous clinical staff (all specialists, all primary care)	Diverse clinical staff (disciplines integrated)
Reputation-based medicine	Evidence-based healthcare
Fee for service	Performance-based compensation
Limited or lack of performance review	Regular review/measurement by peers/patients
Innovation based on individual initiative	Innovation encouraged system-wide mistakes basis of critical learning
Cost-based practice	Affordable, effective, efficient total healthcare

Seven Losses of Physicians

1. Loss of control
2. Loss of income
3. Loss of respect
4. Loss of productivity
5. Loss of joy
6. Loss of identity
7. Loss of autonomy

Learning Disabilities in Healthcare

- Fragmentation
- Polarization
- Fear of future
- Suspect relationship with the community
- Turnover of staff
- Too much management, not enough leadership
- Medical Arms Race
- Destructive internal competition
- Reactive behaviors at all levels
- Split between administrators and physicians

Executive Summary

"Healthcare is unraveling" exclaimed a respondent to healthcare survey. "Not so," said another. "It's already unraveled. In fact, it's broken!"

Based on extensive, broad research, this report addresses three critical questions:

1. **Where have we been in healthcare?**
2. **What's happening in healthcare today?**
3. **What are the critical strategies for the future?**

These questions are explored in the three years study with participants from 48 states.

Participants in the research have suggested that the current disarray and dysfunction and dis-eased state of healthcare systems in the United Sates is the direct result of the confused leading the gullible, that is, executive leaders who know how to create financial forms while knowing little about how to read medical charts are leading physicians and the public down the path of fiscal irresponsibility and threatening to disembowel what has been the finest healthcare delivery system in the world. The United States is no longer the finest healthcare system in the world.

The spin-off of this dysfunction is:

1. **Ten learning disabilities in healthcare**
2. **Seven losses of physicians**
3. **Eleven paradigm shifts impacting healthcare delivery**

The data gathered during this three year research project involved interviews with 511 physicians, physician executives, system administrators, regulators, and third party payers. 117 patients were interviewed and 213 healthcare systems and 9 medical schools constitute the people and system background for the study.

Unraveling and Re-Birth

The research indicates that both the public together with physicians are re-evaluating nearly everything: medical plans, revenue streams, patient expectations and demands, rationing, and the viability of healthcare systems to sustain long term health protection.

The research surfaces practical proposals to deal with the bunker mentality within healthcare, the polarizations within and between systems, a fixation on the fix-it mentality, and the problem that doesn't want to go away, namely, the high cost of healthcare.

The preponderance of evidence gained from the research suggests that there is a serious lack of thinking about leadership, focusing especially on building a vibrant organization and system for the long term. This involves senior executives having a leadership architecture mind-set that links personal, professional, and organizational realities throughout the system as a whole.

The idea of rebirth emerges primarily from the indomitable spirit of Americans who refuse to settle for second best and whose history of rising to challenges is documented in nearly every aspect of our history and development.

While the idea of rebirth is loaded with social, even religious, overtones, the intent of championing the idea emerges from healthcare practitioners and patients who are shouting, even threatening, from every patient room, living room, board room, and break room: WE'RE NOT GOING TO TAKE IT ANYMORE! The public is no longer gullible. The public is more informed, more demanding, and more insistent that excellence can be achieved, and that universal accessibility and coverage is not a potential economic nightmare.

This book is a serious introduction meant for anyone interested in more than debate or positional dialogue. It's an invitation to a focused conversation which, hopefully, will go beyond fixing broken infrastructures and will heal our divisions and put a new heart within us. The philosophical outlook of the rebirth is supported by practical suggestions.

Unraveling, unraveled, renewal. Past, present, and future. The reader is invited to listen to the stories and yearnings of providers, physicians, administrators and patients who want only the best healthcare possible.

Grounded in facts, the study provides a framed focus for the future and suggests that what has unraveled is the prelude to a new future grounded in hope.

Begun as a research project and not to establish or promote one theory of healthcare, leadership, or management as being singularly outstanding, this report is just that, a report which purports to inspire us to take action to improve the health of our nation, our communities, ourselves.

A sequel to this book will address the critical issues uncovered in *Unraveling and Re-Birth of Healthcare* is being prepared by Zobius Leadership International.

Chapter One

The Changing Landscape of Healthcare

Dr. Harry P. Volin conducted his rural medical practice in two rooms in the Exchange Bank in the small town of Lennox, South Dakota. The country was still in the grips of the Great Depression on that hot August day when he delivered the Hoffman twins in their parents' rented house. Edward Hoffman, first-time father employed by the WPA (Works Progress Administration), asked, "What do I owe you, Doc?"

"Do what you can when you can, Ed." Dr. Volin never sent a bill or asked for a dime. In payment Ed gave him 50 cents a month for about two years. The townspeople, including the Hoffmans, kept the Volin larder full of garden produce until their medical bills could be paid in full. That's the way it was.

The twins were a surprise. No technology or procedure existed to predict multiple births. For critical cases only, the low-tech hospital in Sioux Falls was 20 rutted miles from the Hoffman home. Ambulance service in Lennox consisted of Dindot Funeral Service's hearse.

The little town had its own healthcare resources and specialists at that. For a broken hip, the bone expert at hand was Ethel, the post office clerk. Miriam in the hardware store could always help with a difficult baby. For the elderly neighbor wandering disoriented about town, there was Carl in the lumberyard. No directory announced who could do what; there were no fee schedules, no association meetings.

The crude communications functioned most efficiently. Cora, chief telephone operator and principal triage officer, had her ear on everything. We would pick up the phone, give the handle a turn, and enlist her help in all sorts of arrangements. "Cora, this is Jim. Do you know if Harry's in town today? We need some help at the Helmstad farm."

"I'll get on it, Jim," she would say. "I think Harry is out, but Jonas can help. I'll give him a call."

The town itself was the social caretaker, functioning as an American Association of Retired Persons (AARP), a nurses' association, an HMO, and a chief financial group. Its churches connected and

11

mobilized the people of Lennox. The pastors and priest served as official spokesmen for the community. Meanwhile, *The Lennox Exchange*, the weekly newspaper, provided all the detail anyone wanted to read and sometimes more.

A New Era

The end of World War II introduced a new era. Highway 19 was leveled and paved. Suddenly it was much easier to drive to the clinics and hospitals in Sioux Falls. Several clinics installed the kind of on-site diagnostic equipment that could reduce or eliminate patients' hospital stays, a bold move that threatened the role of the hospitals. Some physicians could see that the future of their practice lay in the community clinic rather than in the city hospital. A few physicians observed that hospitals would have to focus on those patients with life-threatening illnesses and those in need of acute care.

The public still held physicians in very high regard. Other than for the grossest neglect or incompetence, a patient did not consider suing a physician. There was no talk of high premiums for malpractice insurance and the cost of medical care was still within most people's reach.

Doctor Volin retired. A primary care physician from a Sioux Falls clinic now spent two days a week in the new Lennox Clinic, a satellite of a Sioux Falls practice. Serious cases in the outlying areas were referred for diagnosis and treatment to the main clinic. The Sioux Valley, McKennan, and VA hospitals continued to serve a large area including South Dakota, southwestern Minnesota, and northwestern Iowa. The concept of managed care had not arrived.

Until 1945 or so, professional providers delivered adequate health care, without explicit concern for capacity or quality, to those who requested it. During the 50s and 60s, concern for healthcare capacity, expanded access, and quality became pronounced among providers and then users as well.

New language reflected and shaped these concerns. Providers spoke of capacity issues with management-oriented terms such as "manpower planning" and "manpower development." The Hill-Burton Act of 1964 enabled smaller communities to build hospitals, and they did. No longer did physicians in small communities send their patients 100 miles away for hospitalization. While the increased number of hospital beds offered a short-term advantage for consumers, in the longer term it became a problem for healthcare planners and providers.

Then, the establishment of Medicare introduced a more insidious effect: physicians could easily become lazy or, worse, they could manipulate testing and billing procedures. Some chose to prosper through fraud.

Managed Care

Planning issues and related language continued to shift during the late 60s. More and more attention was given to Medicare and third-party payment procedures. In the 70s increasing emphasis was placed on "utilization review" (UR), "budget control" (BC), and "financial planning" (FP). The terminology and rhetoric of UR, BC, and FP have held sway through the 80s and into the 90s. By the mid-90s, the evolving concept of "managed care" had matured in some parts of the country, particularly in Minnesota where it originated. The healthcare entities that were managed grew in number and extent. Huge systems emerged. A number of nationally based holding companies such as Humana and Columbia came to own and operate hundreds of medical facilities—hospitals, clinics, diagnostic centers, and same-day surgery centers. This collection gave providers greater leverage in purchasing equipment and supplies. Assumed economies of scale have fed the continuing growth and merging among facilities and among companies.

Now, because of merged facilities, people in small towns and rural areas and remote areas ironically struggle once more with access to professional healthcare. Though highways and telecommunication systems are much improved for outlying areas, specialized medical care for many is again distant. Unlike in the 30s, however, there is no Doc Volin operating in two rented rooms over the bank and there is no network of informal healthcare experts in the community.

Why Our Survey, Why This Book

From the patient's point of view, the hole in the heart of today's industrial healthcare complex is the absence of Doc Volin. Instead of the known, trusted, accessible doctor at the center of medical care there is a kind of void. The pieces and patches of care that people receive cannot add up to a sustained relationship with a key human being in an integrated service system.

The role of doctors has changed as radically as any other aspect of healthcare in the last 50 years. People perceive physicians very differently today from how they saw them just a few decades ago. Physicians perceive themselves very differently.

These are some of the observations that led to our study. We consider physicians to be, without a doubt, the key to the whole prospect and potential of healthcare, whatever its systems. Not only do we believe that physicians must take the lead in changing the system for the better, we're convinced that *only* physicians, acting in partnership with the other players, can change it for the better. Physicians who are "other centered" vis a vis, "self-centered" will emerge as the leaders necessary for the re-birth of healthcare.

In the study basic to this book we surveyed 511 physicians, healthcare administrators, and 117 patients from 213 healthcare systems in the United States in order to elicit the thinking and doing among physicians and other healthcare professionals (see survey, Appendix). We asked about their reasons for entering the profession. We probed their memories of key historical events affecting the practice of medicine. We wanted to get a sense of how physicians feel about being physicians and how they want to act upon those feelings. Their action is crucial. The contributors to this book are calling upon physicians to act in accordance with the best and oldest values inherent in the profession, those rooted in the Hippocratic Oath.

The Changing Medical Profession

Why do individuals enter the medical profession? Why do they now, why did they in earlier times, why might they in the future? Our survey revealed certain patterns of responses associated with physicians of different eras. During the first half of this century, individuals entered medical school in most instances because they were motivated to become caring healers of other individuals. For them, medicine was a kind of direct calling similar to that of clergy.

Reasons for entering the profession during the 50s and 60s were more layered. A desire to serve the community as a healthcare provider with a strong social conscience was common. In the 70s and 80s compensation, prestige, and scientific orientation became more explicit attractions. Now, in the 90s, the profession appears to be attracting many caring, competent individuals who, once again, feel called.

During these periods, increasingly sophisticated technologies, together with ongoing social change, have reoriented the way we think about work in the U.S. and created new forms of entitlement and accountability. Doctors have not been immune to the influence of such changes or of the social positioning of their own specific generation.

Unraveling and Re-Birth

Differences among their generations have affected their changing outlooks.

On the basis of their belief that history creates distinctive generations and distinctive generations create history, William Strauss and Neil Howe classified the generations of this century.[1] The authors characterized people born between 1883 and 1900 as cautious individualists who came to be known as the *Lost Generation*. Those who arrived between 1901 and 1924, the *GI Generation*, launched America into an expansive era of material affluence, global power, and civic planning. Then came the *Silent Generation*, born 1925-1942. The narcissistic Baby Boom Generation, 1943-1964, who asserted the primacy of self and challenged the moral vacuity of the time's institutional order, disrupted the relative conformity of this group. The relatively neglected Generation X, 1961-1981, followed these indulged Boomers literally the 13th generation to call itself American. Sometimes referred to as "Generation Y," the next generation emerging is another story.

Nearly fifty million Americans were born to the Silent Generation in America between 1925 and 1942. Before them were the so-called G.I. Generation and after them the Boom Generation, then the X, and now the Millennial.

The Silents brought us civil rights, an unparalleled national wealth in the arts and (of course) in commerce, and unimaginable advances in science and technology.

1956:	Early boomers ten years old; late boomers are eight years away from birth. Meanwhile President Eisenhower wins re-election, and Nikita Khrushchev says, "History is on our side. We will bury you!"
1957:	The Russians launch Sputnik I and Sputnik II; President Eisenhower uses troops to enforce desegregation in Arkansas.
1958:	The U.S. launches the Explorer I satellite; the first Pizza Hut opens.
1959:	Barbie is "born"; Buddy Holly dies; Castro takes over in Cuba.
1960:	The soviets shoot down a U.S. spy plane; John Kennedy is elected president; and Chubby Checker introduces the Twist.
1961:	The Russians and then the U.S. put a man into space; the Berlin wall goes up.
1962:	K-Mart and Wal-Mart open; Russian warheads in Cuba bring the world to the edge of war.

1963:	President Kennedy is assassinated; Dr. Martin Luther King declares, "I have a dream."
1964:	President Johnson declares a "war on poverty," ushering in the "Great Society."
1965:	Civil disturbances over race and the Vietnam war play in increasingly larger roles in American society.
1966:	The Supreme Court issues its "Miranda" ruling; U.S. troop strength in southeast Asia reaches 400,000.
1967:	The first heart transplant operation is performed; race riots kill dozens in Detroit.
1968:	Dr. Martin Luther King and Bobby Kennedy are assassinated; President Johnson declines to run for re-election; Richard Nixon wins the presidency.
1969:	The U.S. lands a man on the moon; teens celebrate at Woodstock, then demonstrate in Washington.
1970:	Campus demonstrations close down several colleges; four are killed at Kent State University.
1971:	The "Pentagon Papers" are published; President Nixon freezes wages and prices.
1972:	President Nixon wins re-election in a landslide; the break-in at the Watergate seals his fate.
1973:	The military draft ends; the Supreme Court legalizes abortion.
1974:	Richard Nixon resigns; President Ford declares, "Our long, national nightmare is over." The youngest of the boomers are nearly teenagers; the oldest are nearly middle aged.
1975:	"The Greatest" retains his title in "The Thrilla' in Manila"; Saigon falls and the U.S. bails out of Vietnam; "Jaws" scares the living daylights out of us.

In turn, the different generations from which our physicians have come were shaped by historical events and related changes in society and its values. The following telegraphic list of key events from the years 1920 to 2001 forms a backdrop for the U.S.'s changing approach to healthcare and the medical profession.

1921	Legalization of cigarettes in Iowa
1923	Founding of first birth control clinic: New York City
1928	Discovery of penicillin
1940	U.S. population of 131,669,275
1945	Addition of fluoride to water supply for widespread prevention of tooth decay: Grand Rapids, Michigan
1948	Kinsey Report on male sexual behavior

Unraveling and Re-Birth

1949	Cortisone discovered
1950	US population now 150,697,000
1954	Distribution of Salk's polio vaccine in the U.S
1954	First testing of oral contraceptives for women
1960	FDA approval of "the pill," Enovid
1960	Recognition and treatment of hypertension; Development of chlorthiazide, Diuril, by Merck; Increase in funding for National Institute of Health
1962	Birth of thalidomide-deformed babies in Europe
1964	Hill-Burton Act Establishment of Medicare
1966	Cult of LSD as led by Timothy Leary; First sex change operation in U.S.
1967	US population of 200 million
1967	First human heart transplant, performed by Dr. Christian Barnard
1976	Legal right to stop life support systems achieved by parents of Karen Ann Quinlan
1977	The "end" of smallpox in the world
1978	Birth of first baby conceived in test tube
1979	Publication of Masters and Johnson research exploding myths about heterosexual and homosexual behavior
1990	Break in gene code Identification of AIDS epidemic Emergence of resistance to antibiotics among micro-organisms
1993	Total of 31,279 people waiting for compatible donor organs: 23,533-kidneys; 2,843-hearts; 2,645-livers; 1,071-lungs;140-pancreases; remainder-both kidney, pancreas or heart, lungs
1994	Mergers of 650 hospitals
1996	74% of all enrollments in the country's HMOs accounted for in seven HMOs
1996	Health food a $6.2 billion industry
1997	Cloning of sheep (Dolly) and cattle
2001	Plan to clone humans in place

Although our 20th century played itself out with unspeakable brutality, it ended with some scientific and political triumphs. We are, overall, healthier. People live much longer than during any previous age. We have more open and extended communications than ever. We benefit from new technologies that are developing more rapidly than ever before. In many places and spaces, we have moved away from competition to cooperation.

What are we learning about the practice of medicine over this technologically intense history? We're learning, simply, that **medical practice still requires a personal touch that patients still want to speak with their physicians, and that charts, reports, and pictures cannot replace a doctor.** We're learning that bigger is not necessarily better, that patients do not relate to systems; the relationship is with nurses and doctors. We're learning that power structures in healthcare organizations gave form to the whole landscape of healthcare as well as to the experience of all its participants.

This foregoing set of learnings mainly reflects the perspective of users looking into the system, pretty much from the outside. There's more to learn from the historical experience of physicians themselves inside the system.

Doctors Remembering the Past

Through their own experience, most of our contributors and survey respondents are able to recall and document the changes that have shaped medical history since World War II; some even remember World War I. They share memories of the key events, including those listed above, that affected the professional training and development of physicians.

They recall the 40s and 50s as the onset of the antibiotic era. At this time also we were just beginning to recognize hypertension as a problematic condition. By 1944, President Franklin Roosevelt's blood pressure had risen to 300/170 from a 1934 reading of 136/80. Today we gasp at such numbers and understand that blood vessels will rupture under that kind of pressure. It was inevitable that Roosevelt would die from a cerebral hemorrhage. Yet, when it occurred, news headlines quoted the president's personal physician, Admiral Ross, to say, "It came out of the clear blue sky!"

Hypertension and its complications came to be identified in the 60s and 70s as the leading cause of death. The first effective medication—Chlorthiazide, marketed as "Diuril" by Merck—was not always used properly. For many it proved a lifesaver. In retrospect, this period emerges as Stage I of a burgeoning medical marketplace.

Advances in the 80s allowed medicine to salvage people stricken with myocardial infarctions. Previously, those patients were given a hypo and put to bed with the hope they would still be around in the morning. Then the idea arose that lidocaine, a medication used for many years as a local anesthesia, would decrease myocardial irritability. By reducing the irritability of the heart muscle and subsequent abnormal and fatal heart rhythms, this old medication in its new role lowered the death rate from heart attacks by 50%.

Access to and payment for such medical care options had been largely egalitarian in the 70s, without regard to patients' various funding sources. A new effect crept into the system when some insurance companies, eager to develop a network of insured physicians, attracted and enrolled doctors with a new carrot. They showed that doctors could raise their fees if a company insuring more income held the policies they chose. The related cost plus billing procedure came to be characterized as the "open checkbook" effect.

Rapidly increasing knowledge and technology supported sub specializations and more rationale for higher fees. In response to both medical advances and increased variation in fees, cost controls arrived, HMOs emerged, and closed panel medical plans were formulated. While physicians were still regularly consulted about the impact of medical technology, HMOs were making the administrative decisions regarding the physicians' practice. Increasingly, physicians were being managed more than led, and their discontent became apparent. We had passed into Stage II of the medical marketplace.

During the early 90s, explosive improvement in diagnostic technology and methods took a lot of guesswork out of medical practice. No longer could a doctor say, as I remember an older physician exclaim many years ago, *"I don't know what's wrong with you, but I will operate and find out."* Given new scanning techniques, surprises during surgery are now rare. Physician input has been playing a smaller and smaller role in the technologically intense, corporate environment of healthcare.

Meanwhile, mega-mergers, monopolies, increasingly managed medical care brought reduced options for patients (e.g., little access to physicians, specialists, and treatments of choice). Varying payer systems became more efficient for insurance companies, while complicating the delivery of medical care. Physicians had difficulty with "efficient" medicine; their discontent became more vocal. We had entered Stage III of the medical marketplace.

Some economists still classify the late 90s as Stage III; a new structural effect may introduce another stage. Currently, employers are trying to establish a defined and fixed structure of benefits, thereby making consumers responsible for the level of care purchased. This movement could lead to possibilities for greater user choice, in specific markets; it is unclear if such a change would resolve any of the greater inefficiencies. At any rate, I would call this kind of non-systemic tinkering Stage IV.

Into the Present

Discontent with many aspects of healthcare management and delivery has been growing among various constituencies, including certainly that of physicians. The public in general is becoming more interested in and more aware of such findings on physicians as the following:
- Of physicians we surveyed, 40% would choose not to go to medical school if they had it to do it over again.
- The incidence of disability due to physical accident, emotional stress, and medical impairment among physicians has risen 35% since 1993. (Medical Economics: 8/01)
- The frequency and cost of individual claims have both shot up 60% since 1994. (Medical Economic: 7/99)
- Disgruntled patients' complaints to the Boards of Medical Registration have doubled in the past five years and continue to increase by 20% per year. (Archives: Medical Economics)
- The U.S. has a surplus of 150,000 physicians today. Bureau of Primary Health Care, Health Resources and Services Administration, US Dept. of Health and Human Services
- Among graduating physicians we surveyed, 10% can't find jobs in their specialties.

The medical professional appears to be unraveling. Many consumers, physicians, allied staff, and healthcare professionals disagree with this assertion, claiming that it has already unraveled.

Our research indicates, not surprisingly, that the depth of physicians' caring about patients varies: it goes up when work and income are plentiful, and down when patient load increases and income decreases, and when patient load decreases along with income. While some managed care providers and physicians care less overall about the individual patient, is there any constituency who cares more? Wall Street and insurance companies are interested in patients only to the extent that patients are the occasion for their enterprises and profits. Is all this a quandary for patients, physicians, or both? Both.

Until recently in historical terms, quality care and strong physician-patient relationships formed the Hippocratic foundations of professional healthcare as well as of embryonic healthcare systems. Even scientific advances in the diagnosis, the understanding, and the treatment of illness were due to physicians' motivation and ingenuity. Now, the times present an extremely complex work environment for physicians. They can't simply go back to an earlier, simpler one. Physicians must become wisely adept in today's environment no matter what their mission, even and especially if they wish to take on a wholesale transformation of our healthcare system.

Doctors Acting Wisely

The people who have been managing and changing the role of physicians are not physicians themselves, nor necessarily persons who understand physicians or their work. Just to deal effectively with these critical stakeholders, doctors have to develop new sets of skills they've largely ignored in their long quest for initial and ongoing professional training and development. They also must become acquainted with the whole range of critical healthcare issues in addition to their own immediate concerns, and be willing to take them on.

Currently, the fundamental objectives affecting that whole range of issues are containing costs and meeting patient demands, objectives that obviously conflict with one another. Widely publicized technological advances and advertising by companies producing healthcare related products ratchet up patient expectations quickly. At the same time, ultimate stockholders in healthcare corporations want earnings, the more the better, even though some of these same individuals are likely to be patients demanding the latest, most expensive medical interventions themselves. This Gordian knot needs a lot of bright, imaginative people to untie it, including in particular well-educated, well-informed, business-savvy physicians.

On the cost-containment end, physicians should be able to work with other healthcare professionals and the greater society to eliminate unnecessary demand for and use of services, and to continuously reduce healthcare costs through quality management on every front. Physicians need to persuade people of the longer-term savings in both money and personal health that can be achieved by solid preventive strategies (e.g., early detection and treatment of disease, the elimination of tobacco and other drug usage). Further, **physicians better than anyone else can attest to the counterproductive pile-up of non-uniform administrative procedures multiplying in both healthcare provider organizations and insurance companies.**

Physicians are busy professionals. It takes some learning to become savvy in a business "system" drifting further and further away from our comprehension of it. Where do doctors even begin to become adept, to develop the business perspective they need to become serious players in this environment? There are starting points.

Doctors need to understand clearly that they are dealing with many stakeholders in addition to patients. They need to know who the critical healthcare stakeholders and players are and, eventually, whether as individuals or professional units, to form working relationships with all of them. Ultimately, they need to go into non-medical environments to consult on critical healthcare related issues, while confidently speaking the language of finance, insurance risk coverage, and technical engineering. Physician executives must master the basics of effective communications with all stakeholders.

It would behoove HMOs to foster managerial and executive leadership in their own physicians through targeted training and development. These organizations need to see that as long as physicians feel marginalized in their own profession they will consider organizing themselves for the same ends of greater participation in the management and decision making of the corporation.

Transitions and the Next Fifteen Years

In our survey, we asked members of the medical community for their thoughts on where we are now regarding healthcare and where we're going in the future with it. What approaches and strategies might we enlist to change the current situation? What forms could/will healthcare take?

In considering its past and imagining its future, none of the respondents appears to have forgotten the patient as the reason for healthcare. The respondents are at the same time familiar with a spectrum of stakeholders and their basic interests. **To physicians, healthcare is an occupation, an opportunity to help and heal, and a means to earn an income.** To investors it's a chance to be part of the fastest growing industry in America, and a means to increase income.

To Wall Street it's a business with considerable potential, and a means to increase income. To society, healthcare is a service to individuals that can improve the overall health of the community. To patients it's a necessity, a safety net in good and bad times, and without patients, there can be no healthcare industry. Patients are the real bottom line and physicians apparently understand that point. In order for the rebirth of healthcare to become authentic, more than a safety net will be required. A wholistic system centered on community health rather then illness will be necessary for the optimization of healthcare.

Patients: The Past and Future Bottom Line

While we are all individual patients or potential patients/users of healthcare, it is natural for us as to want healthcare without boundaries for ourselves. In business terms, boundaries are needed for control, cost-effectiveness, and confidentiality. Nonetheless, boundaries set to protect the system rather than serve the patient need to be redrawn or eliminated.

A focus on patients means more than customer service. Instead of being a distraction to the booming enterprise of healthcare, as we may sometimes feel, we patients must be central to every budget generated, every needle manufactured, every chart completed, every person employed in the industry, every brick laid in the facilities, every CAT scan administered, every training session organized, and every merger contemplated.

Administrators and physicians are quick to point out privately that the soul of healthcare is being contaminated by greed. That they refer to a soul is good news. Whatever that soul consists of, it's associated with a Hippocratic tie between the caregiver and cared for. The patient is not only the anchor to the system, the patient is the unchanging point of reference for transition and change in healthcare. There will be new diseases, new DRGs (diagnostic resource group), new treatment procedures, new medicines, new technologies. Doctors anticipate a great deal of change in the practice of medicine and very little change in human needs and expectations. At their most optimistic, they believe that high tech *and* high touch can and will shape the future of healthcare.

Toward Wellness

Implicit in our respondents' vision is a welcome humility in the face of our advances. Moreover, any discussion of the future involves some notion of probabilities and some exercise of intuition, best informed by knowledge of the past. We're all becoming more aware that a basic shift in emphasis from treatment to wellness is occurring in our overall approach to healthcare. Healthcare providers must change their primary mode of thinking from treatment to wellness.

People do not want to get sick or be sick. The stress, growing among consumers as well, is on prevention. A physician skilled in nuclear medicine has issued a related warning to people taking on their own preventive care:

Patients are becoming more informed about wellness. Noticing the rapid growth of health clubs and exercise parlors confirms that idea that the people want to be healthier. However, there are areas where the public can be misled and physicians can correct these false ideas. For example, some diet fads can be dangerous, even fatal. Some health programs can be extremely costly and worthless. Sometimes it's important that physicians speak up, tactfully.

It's important to recognize that non-establishment interventions (e.g., interventions herbal, homeopathic, or other "alternative medicine") are more often castigated by doctors than many equally or more problematic establishment (e.g., serious to fatal prescription drug reactions).

New Treatment Configurations

With growing stress on prevention in both establishment and non-establishment medicine, treatment strategies need to be reconfigured for both greater economies and improved patient care. One model of innovative treatment facilities is the Sinai ER-7 Emergency Center in Baltimore. Built from the ground up to set new standards of rapid-response patient care and customer service, ER-7 takes a dramatically different approach to care. It has seven specialized emergency centers under one roof.

Its **Fast Track** facility offers ready care to patients with minor ailments such as sprains, sore throats, and small cuts. It allows patients with less critical conditions to receive the immediate attention normally reserved for patients with more critical conditions.

Urgent Care is a unit equipped for dental, ear, eye, nose and throat emergencies; the unit has a specially and creatively designed gynecological obstetric examination rooms complete with a private adjoining restroom; and an orthopedics room offering advanced techniques in pain management techniques for patients with broken bones or fractures.

Emergent Care provides intensive care and individual monitoring for critically ill patients. Its special elevator transports critically ill patients to operating rooms or an intensive care unit with a full range of equipment for patients' critical needs. All private rooms feature glass walls that face the nurses' area, allowing both constant supervision and privacy.

The **Trauma Center** is an immediate-response unit staffed by a specially trained trauma team that provides life-saving care. It is equipped with rapid resuscitation and CT scanning, and is designed with a variety of entrances to receive patients from ground transportation or from helicopters that land on a rooftop helipad.

Pediatrics Care Center provides emergency care for children in a cheerful environment that makes a young patient's emergency room experience as positive as possible. It offers full-time pediatric physicians and nurses. It includes full-time play areas.

The **Chest Pain** evaluation center is an advanced cardiac care program that features an extensive monitoring system, an ambulance-to-hospital EKG transfer system, advanced cardiac stress tests, and an evaluation unit for individuals experiencing chest pain without evidence of a heart attack.

Observation Center serves individuals whose medical conditions require extended evaluation and/or treatment. It allows patients to be monitored on an outpatient basis instead of being admitted to the hospital. Each glass-enclosed room features a television and special, comfort-designed bed. Large windows offer observation visibility without sacrificing patient privacy.

The **Sinai ER-7** healthcare center addresses different levels of patient needs efficiently. Its configuration of ready, effective service meets customer needs. At the same time, its specialized facilities are designed wisely from a management point of view. These Baltimore facilities respond in many ways to what people want in their healthcare services.

Listening to Patients

In addition to their growing desire for both wellness and for responsive treatment options when they need them, ordinary people in the U.S., I believe, have some basic concerns that are disturbingly reflective of how far we have to go. We hear a lot of the following kinds of comments:

- Healthcare is changing and I don't like it.
- My doctor used to know me personally and care about me.
- Healthcare is more expensive than I can manage and it scares me.

Prior to setting policies and establishing long-term strategies, healthcare providers and planners need to become more aware of the mind-set of ordinary people, average citizens, and the whole range of patients—the people who employ them in effect and on whose behalf healthcare professionals earn their livelihoods. Healthcare strategies in the U.S. tend to get set in stone quickly, irrespective of what patients think, feel, or want. This public-be-damned attitude is arrogant, dishonorable, and deserving of quick rejection. The wellness of healthcare itself depends upon a public-be-served attitude.

Not only do individual doctors need to learn to listen to individual patients, the whole industry needs to listen to patients. Consider the questions below with direct reference to your own "patient" point of view. (Think of the cardiologist who saw a totally different world of healthcare when he himself became a long-term patient and then wrote a book about the horrors of that world.)

- How do you know if your vision of healthcare is ailing or healthy, distorted or accurate?
- How do you measure the health of the industry, and why?
- What perspectives, insights, and criticisms are you hiding in your organization?
- What difference would it make if you were not a part of the policy-making table?
- What drives your organization? Is it money, the past, power, competition, habit, other?

HMOs are not universal. In addition to consumers, many journalists and healthcare critics view HMOs as an abysmal failure. HMO executives are aware of the challenges of capitation and the increasing dissatisfaction and demands of the public. A rush to judgment regarding the health of all HMO organizations is unwarranted.

HMOs, hospitals, clinics, and other healthcare delivery organizations all have a future. How can an HMO make an important contribution without first changing its structure and mission radically? And who will figure out its fit? Rebels, often seen as "subversives" who break the rules and take risks, create the most innovative futures. Doctors are not necessarily risk-averse. Some are risk takers and some are not.

Multiple Strategies

To cut through the complexities of today's medical industrial complex means taking on and integrating multiple strategies. One such strategy is the pilot program, a kind of sampling technique. The sample does not tell everything, too often not enough. Sometimes it's as naive as the blindfolded person touching the leg of the elephant and calling it a tree trunk, and sometimes it's as profound as DNA testing. There's no risk-free sample; the small-scale pilot approach can help lay foundations for lasting, managed change. Statistical sampling and piloting techniques is key to quality management methods, forming the basis for thoughtful, informed improvement in the system.

Over the decades, healthcare has regressed and progressed, seeming to swing between regression and development. Some strategies and attempts at systemic change and improvement will backslide. Creativity is needed right off just to imagine effective approaches and strategies to change.

Before plotting and planning change in your organization or in the industry at large, dare to dream and get others—all kinds of healthcare practitioners plus all kinds of patients—to do the same. Imagine how, with the advanced medical and communications technologies we have, healthcare could work in the most wonderful ways for doctors and patients. Wonderful things in healthcare are within our reach. Some are already happening:

In Jordan, kings and citizens alike can receive medical care from physicians at the Mayo Clinic in Minnesota. King Hussein has his checkups through a satellite link that bounces images of blood vessels, chest X-rays, and ultrasound records, while he and his Mayo-based doctor discuss how he has been feeling. Jordanian physicians will also be educated by satellite from their Mayo colleagues on breast cancer, heart rhythm, and malignancies. The Mayo Clinic now plans other international links to Greece and possibly Argentina, Chile, and Colombia. –

Minneapolis Star & Tribune 9/2000

Chapter 2wo

Unraveling Chaos

Many expert attempts to improve healthcare today have been counterproductive. Experts continue to address discrete parts of the problem without a vision of the whole, and over time the solutions exacerbate the problem. Meanwhile the chaotic empire of healthcare continues to sprawl like the American megalopolis. As new, separate suburbs spread throughout the metropolitan area without coordinated planning or oversight, the sectors of the medical industrial complex spread without central management.

The huge systems in which we live and work are fluid and ever changing. Sooner or later a system will lose its synchrony and need some creative thinking and doing to keep it healthy. Localized and surface problems can signal deeper, more pervasive problems. Too often we leap to repair the conspicuous glitch and fail to look deeper for its root cause. We waste energy pointing fingers, fixing blame, and then apply a quick fix, a bandage. We do that in politics, government, marriages, corporate organizations, in city management, and in healthcare. **Repeatedly we fail to solve the problems we identify, compound the ones we haven't identified, while draining our energy and becoming defensive and disillusioned.**

Like the systemic problems facing us, our attempts at resolution should be multifaceted. We need to identify what is working and why in our healthcare system so that we can support the positive and better address what is not working and why. We must make adept choices intellectually in the chaos of healthcare today with an openness and agility to pursue deeper order and disorder in the system. A seeker of deep solutions to deep problems takes the long view and, when caught in an organizational sand trap, says, "This sand trap presents a remarkable challenge. Let's focus on what needs to be done."

"No great improvements in the lot of mankind are possible until a great change takes place in the fundamental constitution of their modes of thought," said John Stuart Mill. From Heraclitus to Thomas Kuhn, wisdom of the ages gives us similar advice. To heal healthcare, we need to problem-solve across the boundaries of its issues, the

Unraveling Chaos

functions of its varied professionals, and the interests of its stakeholders. It's important for us to understand the history of healthcare in this country to see how we got to where we are, not to place blame for our present situation. The very nature of healthcare lays in problem solving, in analytic diagnosis with treatment for, when best, the whole patient.

Now is the time to celebrate our successes and to create a new future with new solutions. Physicians need to lead the way. Well-trained, often brilliant professionals, physicians may dislike the responsibilities and processes of management and they certainly dislike being managed. Nonetheless, they possess some powerful management skills: they know how to examine problems and base decisions on data and experiential learning.

While doctors have strong skills that they can transfer to the problem solving and decision making required to improve healthcare for all its participants, they may not see their own potential to act as leading agents of change. They may be struck by the management skills they lack. Inexperienced with group processes and consensus building methods, they generally also lack business acumen or savvy. Maybe more immediate roadblocks to leadership, however, are their feelings of discouragement and depression about their loss of autonomy, and the reductions in the respect, status, and income they receive. Some admit to a loss of professional personal identity. For many, the joy of medicine has soured.

The world's best health care? Charlene Johnson's report (Ladies Home Journal, Sept. 2001) is sobering and instructive. She reflects on the World Health Organization's (WHO) assessment of 191 nations, looking at factors such as overall health of the populations and comparing access to healthcare for rich and poor. The results:

The best health system in the world: **FRANCE**
Per capita health-care spending in France: **$2,369**
Worst health-care system in the world: **Sierra Leone**
Per capita health-care spending in Sierra Leone: **$11**
Country that spend the most per capita on health care: **U.S. $4,187**
Where the U.S. health system ranks: **37th place**
Why? The U.S. scores low on access to health care, lifestyle issues such as diet and safety and life expectancy of certain groups.

37th place. More evidence that our healthcare system has unraveled. Healthcare systems are in need of leadership and organizational architecture that will allow re-birth to occur. Healthcare leaders at every level are conflicted about what can and must be done. The fix-it mentality is strong in healthcare; it often takes precedence over examining the realities that are rendering healthcare delivery inept. Wise decisions cannot be made in a fix-it mind set. Systems can learn from the Shalowitz study and perhaps apply these learnings to entire healthcare systems.

According to J. I. Shalowitz (Kellogg School of Management, Northwestern University 1994), physicians pass through seven stages before they feel comfortable enough to accept at-risk contracts within or from a system:

- They're unaware or don't know what you're talking about.
- They deny: I don't believe you. Or, it won't happen here.
- They're angry: If you had run this system right, we wouldn't be in this situation.
- They're conflicted about what to do.
- They're resigned and even accepting: "We don't like it, but we have to deal with it."
- Curiosity begins: I wonder how it might work.
- Finally, acceptance, and they will at least accept some small fee discounts.

Many still may be grieving the death of the good old days, the good old ways of fee-for-service medical practice, and the loss of established doctor-patient relationships. Most physicians, however, are beyond the denial stage of grief and accept that many of the good old ways are gone for good. Their stage of response is real, if unfocused anger.

Others physicians are in a bargaining stage, hoping to work out a deal to keep their fee-for-service practice in return for limited reliance on a third-party payer.

The stages create an emotional roller-coaster ride for doctors moving from fee-for-service to a contract environment, from being an independent provider to a salaried employee. Their individual perspective compounds their dilemma. Widening their perspective to see more points of view might pull them out of the narrowest and discouraging positions.

Unraveling Chaos

What Doctors Have Said

During the past ten years I have worked with more than 500 physicians as a friend, coach, instructor, and interviewer. I have heard complaints, challenges, and celebrations. Their own words (below) reflect the industrial repositioning of doctors that they themselves, to some extent, have acquiesced in. They refer to problems in medical training as well as practice.

- Wall Street controls healthcare now.
- Medicine used to be fun.
- My future is in the hands of the insurance company, especially by some bureaucrat who can't even spell "medicine."
- Administrators are more concerned about cost efficiency than disease prevention.
- Patients used to take us seriously. Now they think we're just trying to take them.
- I'm working twice as hard for less income.
- Medical school did not prepare me for a lot of what I'm doing today.
- I'm drowning in paper work.
- Medicine is coming unraveled.
- I'm on a slippery slope and I'm not sliding up. The slope is likely to end in a rush toward a waterfall.
- Many of us over 50 can't wait to retire.
- My identity used to be clear; who I am isn't clear anymore.
- Medicine is a wonderful profession. Why can't we just practice medicine? Answer? Because we have to manage care.
- I can't keep up. The information explosion is as much a liability as an asset.
- We don't know how to collaborate. We are loose cannons who want patients to come to us. We want to own them and we'll share them only in a medical crisis.
- I learned medicine by disciplines. I memorized and forgot a lot of stuff quickly.
- I practice medicine by disease and not by discipline. Why don't medical schools get active about this serious training deficiency?
- Medical training needs to be both training and education. It's a noble profession and our medical students are being taught by many who do not know how to teach, do not know how students learn and don't understand what the customer needs and wants.

- Report cards. Report cards. I've been getting them for decades. We're being graded all the time. What's the big deal? It's the Doc who gets Cs who's against them.
- Which way will medicine go? Will it go with HMO? Will capitation be devastating since it is not a viable form of reimbursement?
- I'm living somewhere between having total control and total despair. It's like trying to solve a medical Rubik's Cube.
- I would go to medical school again with enthusiasm. When there, I loved the chance to learn actual hard data about the structures and functions and care of human beings.
- The crisis we are facing in organized medicine is a good thing. As physicians, we know how to deal with a crisis. There's little reason to fear the future. We'll apply our best skills. It's in us to do so. However, we must be concerned about incompetence at every level.

Significant shifts in the practice and delivery of healthcare reflected here include:

From	*To*
Primary focus on physician	Focus on patients/partnerships
Teaching medical students	Creating learning environments
Individual focus	Team focus
Discrete disciplines	Inter-disciplinary
Isolated specialties	Integrated practices
Discipline-based practice	Wellness (illness prevention) based practice
Homogenous clinical staff (all specialists, all primary care)	Diverse clinical staff (disciplines integrated)
Reputation-based medicine	Evidence-based healthcare
Fee for service	Performance-based compensation
Limited or lack of performance review	Regular review/measurement by peers/patients
Innovation based on individual initiative	Innovation encouraged system-wide mistakes basis of critical learning
Cost-based practice	Affordable, effective, efficient total healthcare

Unraveling Chaos

Physicians' Seven Significant Losses

We have learned that these changes are difficult for physicians and that there is no end in sight. What was once a stable environment for clinics, long-term care, and hospitals, is now unstable. Unprecedented and unpredictable change—driven by technology, the digital economy, market and other forces—have conspired to reshape just about everything about healthcare. Standing at the center of the new chaos, physicians are feeling the direct reduction or loss of seven attributes that have been crucial to their professional role: control, autonomy, income, respect, identity, joy, productivity. The remainder of this chapter addresses each of these along with some strategies for dealing with them.

Control
Autonomy
Income
Respect
Identity
Productivity
Joy

1. Loss of Control

A physician with more than 30 years of practice in clinical and academic medicine says:

> *Today's doctor has less and less control over the practice of medicine. S/he is working for the HMO and PPO. They may not want the doctor to give full disclosure to the patient, which could result in more testing procedures, which, of course, increases the cost. The physician must be at every negotiation table or be represented by another physician at every negotiation table. To exclude the physician will mean the disintegration of patient care.*

The declaration makes a number of points:

- Now control in medical practice is shared.
- Many physicians are now employees, not independent providers.
- A patient is likely to know less about his/her condition and pay more.

Unraveling and Re-Birth

- Physicians must bargain with payers to care patients and must know when to say *No* to the payer.
- The health of healthcare's future depends on physicians' central role in it.

Physicians believe that healthcare is now in the hands of Wall Street and that Wall Street is happy to be in control. Wall Street seems to have concluded that physicians cannot manage anything and should not have any real control over the future of healthcare. The gloves are on!

Coming to the Table

Wall Street knows how to make and manage money. Physicians know how to diagnose both health and illness and manage the treatment process. Who or what should control the future of healthcare? Is there room for physician, accountant, broker, and insurance company at the same table? If so, who will manage or facilitate the discussion? Who will ensure that strategic thinking occurs? Currently, three separate and non-aligned groups are making strategic plans. Wall Street, acting on behalf of shareholders and stockholders, is planning to merge and purge. Physicians are reacting to their loss of control by threatening unionization and the pooling of resources to buy back institutions. Insurance companies are controlling by capitation.

A physician in practice for more than 20 years writes:

> *Doctors feel a loss of control. There is a dilemma concerning what hospital administrators and managers have to do and what doctors want to see happen. That is creating a great deal of tension. While everyone says that the answer to relieving that tension is collaboration, it's easier said than done. Doctors have diverse personalities, and most meetings set up by management continue to be a pain for doctors. They would rather work one-on-one than sit in a meeting. As long as that sort of behavior continues among physicians, we won't get anywhere.*

In visiting with physicians and healthcare administrators all over the U.S., I've heard only a few physicians use the word "collaboration." The word is as difficult for some physicians to say as their Latin terms may be for non-physicians to say. Both physicians and healthcare administrators, though, readily use the other "C" word—*competition*.

Unraveling Chaos

Seemingly opposites, cooperation or collaboration and competition can fuse, to some degree, in sophisticated negotiations involving game theory strategies. The term given to such efforts is *co-opetition* by management game theorists Adam Brandenburger and Barry Nalebuff. Doctors could benefit from taking such an approach, particularly because the situation is so complex and so fraught with apparently conflicting interests.

Other wisdom offers physicians opportunities to extend their perspectives. A modest quote from Dwight Morrow comes to mind:
> *The world is divided into people who do things and people who get the credit. Try, if you can, to belong to the first class. There's far less competition.*

New Perspectives

Because healthcare is becoming more regionally or nationally controlled, physicians and community leaders fear that commitment overall will be to the system, not to the community or physicians. Seasoned physicians say that, as a profession, medicine needs to refocus on patients and the community. Ideally that refocus would engage systems thinking, and perhaps related chaos or complexity theory.

Systems thinking and complexity theory show that every aspect within a system can affect everything else; nothing stands on its own or can be truly examined, understood, or "integrated" in isolation from the rest of the system. The considerable talk about a need for integrated healthcare is a promise in most areas, not a reality. The difficulty many of us have with systems thinking is that, like economics, it appears to explain everything and predict little. Nonetheless, it will enrich the processes both of problem identification and solution and of decision making immeasurably.

Refocus is needed concerning how managed care organizations can integrate physicians into their management and policymaking. The ability of managed care to manage physicians has peaked. Doctors' growing discontent can energize them to take more control themselves of the way that medicine is practiced. Through a systems approach, they can establish basic partnerships with other stakeholders.

On a larger, public scale, the whole purpose of healthcare needs revisiting. Consumers and professional watchdogs are calling medicine's integrity into question. As a professional class, physicians could be castigated and censured as broadly as lawyers are today. The object here is not a matter of maintaining the integrity of medicine and physicians; the challenge is regaining it.

Language as Key

Physicians have been fractionated by businesses, and some have taken a central role in the business, raising concerns of conflicting interests. To some degree, business has seized or co-opted the roles of organized medicine. Business has its own language, as has medicine, and specialized language can function as an instrument of control. Physicians feel they are being forced to speak the language of business in order to practice medicine. Which language will dominate in our restructuring of medicine, and shape our thinking about healthcare?

The language and processes of such management interventions as "reengineering" are unfamiliar to many in the healthcare community. Further, physicians need to be wary of many management buzzwords and buzz concepts for the confusion and emptiness they can introduce in organizations. Because so many organizations fail to carry out their own promoted programs, good ideas get a bad name. The enormous popularity of *Dilbert* and his daily critiques of management "thinking" is an important indicator of the low success rates of organizational change efforts. Physicians can benefit from management training and from management consultants, and they also need to be aware of the tremendous range in quality among such offerings so that, in their relative naiveté here, they do not waste precious months and years following a hollow call. They need to look at the quality programs that are really working in specific organizations (e.g., Six Sigma at GE, GE Medical Systems, and GE Capital).

Essentially, it is difficult, perhaps impossible, to practice medicine using the bottom-line language of business predominantly, and so consumers and physicians share a common confusion. Prior to the 1970s many consumers had a love affair with medicine, and a love-hate affair with business. Now that business is in bed with medicine, consumers' hearts are bruised, and their love affair with medicine has turned to a love-hate relationship.

I asked a 40-year-old physician in internal medicine, with a Ph.D. in clinical psychology, to discuss the subject of new perspectives for physicians:

> *When we ask these questions of physicians and hear their concerns, their responses don't seem to be thoughtful responses.*

Unraveling Chaos

In fact, all of these issues weigh so heavily on the physician's mind that they leave great dissatisfaction, a dynamic tension, and a sense of losing control over a profession that is theirs. And that's interesting! It depends on where they are in [their careers]. Those who are 55 and older, I think, are just looking to reach the end of their careers and retire. Those who are younger, in medical school—about half of the medical school classes are women—I think have acclimated to a transformed healthcare environment. It's the middle group who are generally the most productive doctors, who are that most dissatisfied, disappointed, and distraught over what's happening in healthcare, especially the economics of healthcare. Many physicians simply do not take the time to do a mid-course correction or think about the future. Most of us hide behind the excuse of time. We tell ourselves that we don't have time; it is a lame attempt to avoid self-confrontation. The future is so scary for most of us that it is easier to complain than to learn a new skill or refocus our internal and physician energies.

The issues this physician/psychologist raises, in my judgment, are best discussed seriously among physicians themselves in a safe environment. The loss of control is not terminal. Doctors can act. They need to come together and be honest with each other about what they want.

2. Loss of Autonomy

Autonomy is the centerpiece of a physician's life and work. The well-used phrase *"herding cats"* is used to describe the difficulty in managing or supervising physicians. Cats are independent and even sacred to many. Throughout much of the Middle- Ages, cats were feared and hated. Because of their nocturnal habits, they were believed to consort with the devil. This association with witchcraft has been responsible for many acts of cruelty toward cats through the centuries. The Renaissance, in contrast, was the golden age for cats. Almost everyone had one, from members of royal families and their staffs to the peasantry.

The first domestic cats in North America arrived with the colonists and were employed to keep the rodent population under Thailand and China.

And so, why this brief venture into the history of cats? Only to note that the history of cats is uneven at best, ranging from objects of the devil to the golden age of deity. Devils and deity are independent, either the object of fear or reverence. It may be time to stop referring to physicians as cats who cannot be organized or as people who do not want to work and live control in the settlers' fields, barns, and homes. Cats are said to have played an important part in keeping rats out of the California gold mines.

In India cats often played an important part in religious or occult ceremonies. In South America the Inca revered sacred cats; cats are represented in pre-Columbian Peruvian artifacts. Cats continue to be worshiped as deities in countries such as together. Stereotyping physicians is as unfair as lumping cats into categories.

A respected physician, who retired at the age of 55, offered another point of view. *"I have always felt a definite discomfort somewhere in side when the phrase "herding cats" is used. I say this because it is fundamentally inconsistent with my experience as a physician leader. It is true that physicians are independent minded and because so many are introverted, they are also psychologically solitary beings. I think that the same can be said of engineers, lawyers, architects and host of other professionals. I see the comment more as something coming from the voice of an 'exasperated control freak' rather than an apt description of physicians. I have found physicians to be people like everyone else. They are smart, have passion and a fair amount of power. People who don't know how to lead comfort themselves with the accusation of "they're cats". I think that it's unfortunate. To put it simply, I see the attribution of "cats" more of a projection than an apt description of Docs."*

The loss of autonomy may be a significant loss if it moves physicians into a collaborative mind-set and environment where cooperation is valued more than competition, where respect for individual contributions is utilized in concert with others.

3. Loss of Income

The most sensitive nerve in the human body is the one that touches the purse. Any discussion of money, income, or the economy has our immediate attention. Our free enterprise system is built on concepts of competition, supply and demand, and market driven goals. Competition presumes there will be a market, and there will be

Unraveling Chaos

contention and opposition played out in it. Exhortations to "take care of yourself first, win!, don't lose whatever you do" represent a kind of ethic that influences so much of our behavior.

What's wrong with that? Who wants to lose? Who wants to be second? What's wrong with the idea of taking care of you first? Right? What patient wants to lose? What patient wants to come in second or have the second team do the surgery? What patient wants the physician to care more about the process than the care? What patient doesn't want the best possible care, no matter the cost?

Money has become a central issue and problem in healthcare today. It may be the central issue that everybody sees in a different way. I remember a story of a mother who sent her two children to the garden. She told the first to bring back as many flowers as she could hold. The second child was told to bring in as many stones as he could hold. When the girl who brought back the flowers, her mother asked, "Did you see the stones in the garden?" No. When the boy returned, the mother asked him, "Did you see the flowers in the garden?" No.

We see what we want to see and what we choose to see. If we look at a patient and see money, the patient becomes an account. If I look at a patient and see a medical need, the patient is a DRG. If I look at a patient and see a person, then I can be a person with another person.

The original model of healthcare was built on the premise that the provider cares for others first, self-second. The notion of competition was not part of the equation. Now, in effect, health care providers are competing with those in need, competing with the sick and injured. Put a vulnerable person in jeopardy for competitive advantage? The language of competition has no place in the healing and caring process. Healthcare must embrace the language of collaboration and cooperation.

When money becomes the prime motivation for healing, healthcare becomes contaminated and potentially paralyzed. Money has become the currency of motivation, achievement and status for many. If we pay peanuts for our highly educated and trained physicians, we'll get monkeys. We are not arguing for low or for inflated incomes for physicians. The argument is for the kind of income that will help cover the immense cost of their medical education and provide for that measure of comfort and pleasure that reduces anxiety, stress, and burden so they can provide high quality medical care and consultation.

The sky is not the limit, neither for the patient or the doctor. Diminishing income is inevitable for today's physician. In the past the charge for a transplant surgery could be as high as a doctor might set it. That is no longer the case, especially with the involvement of the third-party payer.

A survey conducted by the American Medical Association revealed that doctors' incomes are on the rise, reaching nearly $200,000 a year on average in 1996. The report was quick to note that earnings trailed inflation, climbing an average of 2.1 % annually from 1993 to 1996, while inflation rose an average of 2.8 %. That translates into an annual decline averaged over the past three years of .7 %.

Of the physicians we surveyed, 92 % were in practices with managed-care contracts in 1997, up from 88 % in 1996. "There has been a lot of mythology that has grown up around managed care and the impact of managed care on the health care system," says Susan Pisano, spokeswoman for the American Association of Health Plans, representing about 1,000 managed-care plans. "What this data shows is how important it is to look at the facts."

"Quality care takes second place to the bottom line," continues Pisano. Many doctors are seeing more patients while spending less time with them because the aim of managed care, she said, "is to get the most for the least." Physicians can make more money by seeing more patients. That may increase physicians' income; does additional income ensure quality care?

Another physician concerned about providers' relations with pharmaceutical firms was quick to point out that "less access to patients, reduced fee schedules, with resulting decreased income (overhead continues to increase), more restrictions in prescribing practices through the use of formularies all add up to "one of the most disturbing developments in the practice of medicine, with the pharmaceutical companies more deserving of blame than benefits, people, or providers." Many physicians who see the pharmaceutical industry as the pillar of modern medicine offset this comment.

A seasoned urban internist said:

> *Physicians need to accept the fact that we are being paid less although the same expectations of professionalism and performance remain. Physicians are losing income. The surveys can prove almost anything; I'm skeptical about them. Some physicians have lost as much as one-third of the income they reported a decade ago. I know physicians who spend up to three hours daily studying the stock market, managing their portfolios,*

> and comparing notes with brokers all over the world. Managing and making money is the passion for some physicians, and practicing medicine is the job.

Bothered by increasingly negative public perceptions, a 40-year-old primary care physician wrote:

> The perception that all physicians are very wealthy and greedy needs to change. Many of us do not make high salaries. When we need to tell a patient that a service or test is being withheld - because an insurance policy does not permit it - they think we are being greedy. There is a need to change that misperception.

Physicians who take the time to tell patients that some procedures are not necessary or appropriate can change misperceptions. I see what I want to see and choose to see.

4. Loss of Respect

Physicians have lost status and respect. "My son, the doctor…" doesn't have the same weight it long did. Physicians are no longer seen to be at the top of the heap. How do we know this? We asked. A primary care physician speaks for many in his profession:

> We used to matter. Now we might matter. We used to know our patients. If we can't call our patients by name because we know them, we are seen as the guy who changes the oil in our car. I don't care if the quick lube guy knows my name. Just give me the oil and I'll see you in 3,000 miles. Patients want more than that. And we want more than that.

While individual physicians may be self-confident and self-assured, many know that their status in the community has slipped for various reasons, some rational, some irrational. Since it's easier to dismiss an entire population than individuals, individual physicians tend to be more respected than the general population of physicians. A contributing factor to this state of affairs is that few patients have a personal physician. With the possible exception of rural doctors, most physicians no longer have long-term relationships with their patients, and most patients don't have one physician, they have many. If they are fortunate, if they persist and are willing to adjust their schedules, they may see the same physician again and again. The emergence of managed care, together with more demanding medical consumers and a trend toward depersonalization on both ends of the doctor-patient relationship, has resulted in the dethroning of physicians.

No one is free of arrogance. When we ask, "What's in it for me?" we are in a stupid state of arrogance. We are relieved of such stupidity when we change the question to, "What can I do for you?" Unfortunately, arrogant physicians are still with us, though few in number. I suspect that about 10% of all practicing physicians consider themselves to be untouchable, beyond reproach, better than their colleagues, smarter than the smartest. It's not pretty and, more often, it's the arrogant physicians who get sued for malpractice, not open-minded, caring physicians who are able to listen and learn.

5. Loss of Identity

In many states physicians who had been independent contractors with a traditional fee-for-service business model have become employees. No longer legally responsible for running the office, they now report to a vice president of medical affairs or a board of directors. Estimates indicate that over 50% of all physicians in the U.S. no longer sign paychecks, no longer are in charge of their own practice, and have either a dotted or direct line to a corporate executive.

One of our contributors, a medical director of seven nursing homes and also in private practice, observes:

> *Physicians need to figure out how to maintain their identity as physicians while working in a new structure. There is a lot of unrest because physicians are going through a huge change from what they have been used to. They have to operate under the rules and guidelines of managed care.*

When discussing managed care, some physicians roll their eyes and, when pressed, say that it's not managed care, its managed physicians. They admit they don't like management, that they don't like to manage, don't know how to manage, and don't want to learn how to manage.

Yet physicians are being challenged to manage on every front, even if they are operating relatively independently. They have to determine what organizational or corporate structure makes the most sense for their particular practice. They have to manage their own practices in light of rising consumer expectations and possible responses.

A thoracic surgeon has written:

> Physicians have to be much more critical about what is really appropriate care to provide for a patient that will add value to their care. They are dealing with much more scrutiny of their performance from insurance companies, the public, from other physicians. Physicians have to be accountable not only for their ethical conduct, but for quality and efficiency.

Given physicians' changing role and identity, it is a major challenge for them to maintain a high level of professionalism. They may be losing track of how to cultivate a professional career. As employees, they may have less regard for their personal CVs, personal accomplishments, along with a decreased sense of purpose and meaning vis-à-vis the community. Harry F. Halva, a California podiatrist, speaks to the issue of identity:

I Used to Be a Doctor

I used to be a Doctor, now I am a Health Care Provider.
I used to practice medicine, now I function under a managed care system.
I used to have patients, now I have a consumer list.
I used to diagnose, now I am approved for one consultation.
I used to treat, now I wait for authorization to provide care.
I used to cure patients, now I am dared not to cure them by insurance carriers.
I use up the authorization, I lose the patient.

I used to see patients on referral from doctors, patients, and friends, now I must be listed in their Providers Manual.
I used to see patients who traveled to see me, now I am considered out of their approved geographic area.

I used to be paid a Usual, Customary, Reasonable (UCR) fee, now I don't have a usual fee; now there is nothing customary, only managed competition; now who is reasonable?

I used to get paid, now I accept the allowed charges as payment in full for covered services.
I used to be paid for professional services, now I am not paid either for time, materials, or non-allowed services.

I used to be an independent specialist, now I am a dependent ancillary care provider.

I used to provide charity care, now since I am not an authorized provider, I am not permitted to provide charity, or to barter, or to offer advice.
I used to consider the insurance company a third party carrier, now insurance is a fiscal intermediary between the provider and the consumer.

I used to care for patients by appointment, now the patient requires authorization to make an appointment.
I used to provide hands-on care, now I provide hands-off, gloves-on procedures.

I used to use words to describe my care, now I must fill in all the boxes with appropriate code numbers.
I used to provide necessary services, now I am unnecessary.

I used to have a front office coordinator, now triage is performed at the front line.
I used to have a clean office, now I am certified by OSHA.

I used to have a practice, now I am employed to provide services.

I used to have a successful "people" practice, now I have a paper failure.
I used to spend time listening to my patients, now I spend time justifying myself to authorities.
I used to have feelings. Now I have an attitude.

Now I don't know what I am.

6. Loss of Joy

Physicians' work is taxing, exacting, and often exciting. Given the challenges presented by critical illness and the ambiguity of many situations, there is also gratification, contentment, and joy in restoring or maintaining a patient's health, or in becoming genuinely involved with end-stage issues and illness. A senior physician in a clinic of 20 colleagues tells what lessens that kind of gratification and joy:

> The joy of medicine is much less than it used to be. There's more external pressure, more paperwork, less patient contact time. The long-term patient relationships are fewer. If a patient's employer changes insurance companies, you might not be on the new plan. That makes patients and doctors less willing to invest time and effort into their relationship.

The doctor argues that physician or patient satisfaction cannot be achieved without an established physician-patient relationship. This relationship is the linchpin of healthcare, for which the physician makes sacrifices, beginning with training and proceeding through practice. The physician should be rewarded for these basic sacrifices, not overcompensated for certain specialties. Some external pressures need to be alleviated, the doctor continues. Litigation is a problem with a lot of frivolous lawsuits. There should be some reasonable guidelines for litigation, with limitations on fees.

Many physicians are saying that it used to be fun being a Doc. The sadness and resignation behind this declaration are too widespread to ignore. Still, many doctors who are disturbed by the unraveling of medicine on one hand, are cheered on the other hand because it is an opportunity to reinvent the delivery of healthcare and the ways in which illness is dealt with.

7. Loss of Productivity

"Blessed is he who has found his work; let him ask no other blessedness," said philosopher Thomas Carlyle. Physicians are asking in effect to be able to do their work.

They are examining their own productivity and efficacy more and more, wondering if these issues cause that dissatisfaction among the 30% of surveyed physicians who indicate that, if they had it to do over, would not choose to be physicians. Physicians who are troubled or depressed for any reason are less productive than those who are glad to be alive and serving others. Troubled physicians are reactive. A patient presents a problem, the physician reacts. The government presents paper work, the physician reacts. The healthcare system presents policies, the physician reacts. The staff presents demands, the physician reacts. A work life framed by reactive patterns can be depressing, even disabling. Reductions in productivity occur when self-defeating behaviors become trigger responses to common expectations. A disabled physician exhibits one or more of the following counterproductive behaviors: defensiveness; depression; worry; procrastination; compulsivity; smoking; drinking; overeating substance abuse; hostility; perfectionism.

Low productivity is intensified when the physician believes the toxic credo supported by the very medical community in which he or she is a part: If you are anxious, depressed, or even uncomfortable, take medication. Rely on pills. Take your meds. They will get you through the night.

Perfectionist physicians will look for others' approval. Defensive physicians think they are armed against others' feedback. Worrywart physicians feel ready for bad news. Procrastinating physicians feel insulated from making mistakes. Hostile physicians think they look strong. Such self-defeating behaviors are based on mythical, self-deluding fears. How productive can doctors be who are engaged in self-defeating behaviors?

Teflon no longer protects physicians. They are now more exposed than they've ever been. The new ways are not all bad. They need not buckle under the new pressures. Physicians can help and heal themselves. They need to reposition themselves from employee-followers to manager-leaders. This is possible. They can learn to create and maintain linkages and partnerships with a variety of systems, agencies, and individuals in order to practice medicine productively.

Different doctors have different leadership development options. Some physicians can be clinical leaders, while others are capable of both clinical and administrative leadership. Others may emerge as administrative, executive stars. These are natural capabilities that can be developed and refined in medical school and during residency. The current residency program, based on the mentor-coach model, can be developed to include and embed more business-oriented leadership and management training. New partnerships between training institutions and provider institutions can integrate training goals and provide ongoing continuity in learning.

Acknowledging Problems and Developing Trust

Amidst the destructive personal behaviors and organizational entropy that are unraveling healthcare, there are creative forces and opportunities emerging to forge new partnerships among physicians and regulators, patients, and financial/insurance institutions. This is the time to confront fraud in the healthcare system where, according to Malcolm Sparrow, between 20 and 35 percent of the Medicare budget—about $38-63 billion annually—is lost to fraud. *"This is not just sloppy paper work, it's criminal fraud,"* says Sparrow. *"Of the $177.4 billion that Medicare paid to doctors, hospitals, laboratories, and other health care providers in 1997, auditors estimate that about*

Unraveling Chaos

$20.3 billion was wasted." Auditors are not certain about the honest mistakes made in billings and are looking for paper trails in the search for them, the article said.

Education will adapt to these opportunities and become more creative itself. As we prepare medical students for a new and different life in healthcare, instructors will have a new responsibility. Whereas traditional medical education is founded on a teaching model in which they are the experts to whom the students listen, respond, repeat, and replicate, instructors too will have to change their roles. The "teaching" model, effective in the past, is less so now and is changing in some institutions to more of a "learning" model. It's critical that a mentoring model to be in place throughout a physician's career, along with continuous training and development opportunities.

Tied into all the needed openness in training and practice is, of course, the element of trust. The often assumed, fundamental trust between doctor and patient has largely gone the way of their relationship. Today's consumer's greater scrutiny of the doctor should support trust in the enterprise. In some ways, the system is more open to all kinds of scrutiny, acknowledgment of problems, and reasons for various participants to cooperate in taking on challenges. Where they exist, high turnover, lower productivity, and poor morale are evident to all participants. And, ultimately, physicians and healthcare organizations with high levels of distrust have no competitive advantage.

There are reasons for distrust in healthcare organizations. The different players can articulate them. These reasons are not very different from those, which exist in any kind of organization or its management. They include:

- Inconsistency in managerial behavior over time
- Constant change in strategic direction or priorities
- Failure to walk the talk
- Inability to predict behaviors
- Closed or hidden agendas
- Absence of follow-up and follow-through
- Unkempt promises
- Dishonesty
- Unfair treatment regarding conflict, adversity, or failure
- Greater reliability of grapevine than official communications

Unraveling and Re-Birth

In *The Trust Effect*, Larry Reynolds describes eight practices that result in different levels of trust in an organization. The table he provides shows how our organizations measure up.

Practice

1. Choose the right people

Low Trust	Medium trust	High trust
A very slapdash and hurried approach to recruitment	Conventional recruitment of staff-- maybe a couple of one-hour interviews	A very thorough process, which involves at least 12 hours' contact with successful candidate before appointment.

2. Tell them the score

Low Trust	Medium Trust	High Trust
Mission statement, if any, regarded with cynicism	If asked, everyone would give a similar reply to the question "What is this organization for?'	Everyone able to explain how the company as a whole measures success

3. Make them accountable

A lot of blaming others	People have to get permission from their bosses to do things	When something needs to be done, someone does it knowing that the organization will support him or her

4. Identify their concerns

Chief executive never seen	Chief executive has an open-door policy	Chief executive frequently out and about, talking and listening

5. Lead decisively

Staff dissatisfied with the way most decisions are made	Complaints that the managers 'never listen to us' when making decisions	All staff understands how important decisions are reached

6. Act with Integrity

Sloppiness. A promise counts for little. Hypocrisy. Bending the rules	Only a little progress chasing. Meetings start within 10 minutes of advertised time.	Every promise kept. Meetings start and finish on time. People act consistently and ethically.

Unraveling Chaos

7. Give feedback

Low Trust	Medium Trust	High Trust
Lots of talking behind people's backs. Lots of 'office politics'	A company appraisal system which most people find useful	People get frequent feedback from everyone they work with.

8. Promote learning

Not much training or development	Quite a bit of training and development	A big commitment to training and development

People understand these management issues whether they are managers, doctors, administrative clerks, technicians, production workers, and so on. Physicians know a lot more about business and organizational management than they probably think they do. If they could break through a management mystique and take leadership, asserting what they believe to be the best methods of addressing today's problems in healthcare, they could make a giant contribution to the industry and its future.

Chaos and Energy to Go

Sitting over cups of coffee, my wife, Marian, and I were discussing the non-culinary topics of organizational change and chaos. As we talked I played with a pot of water on the stove. As I turned up the flame, the water bubbled and heat rose. I applied more heat, larger bubbles appeared, and there was steam. The hot steam was dissipated as it rose, and the water level fell. Uncontrolled chaos was happening on the stove, energy unbound. When the steam disappeared, its energy was lost. I wondered what could happen if the steam was captured and directed.

Our conversation drifted to healthcare. There's a lot of heat under healthcare and physicians. Some people are getting burned, some are leaving because they can't stand the heat, and all are experiencing the changes.

Physician leaders and key healthcare executives now have the opportunity and the responsibility to recognize the chaos and to capture its energy and power for change. Today's healthcare system is not frozen in stone, by any means. It can continue to change and become something much better for doctors and patients.

Chapter 3hree

Survey and Responses

The survey responses were collected through personal interviews, written responses, and telephone interviews. Approximately 40% of those surveyed represented primary care and internal medicine; 20% were specialists; 30% were physician executives, including CEOs of hospitals or healthcare systems; and 10% were from healthcare administration. Approximately 30% of the total group was women and 8% were African American and first-generation immigrants. Respondents ranged in age from 32 to 70; five of them were retired from medical practice and approximately 5% were within five years of retirement.

The sample was drawn from a diversity of geographic areas, of urban and rural situations, of kinds, ages, and positions of the respondents. For the greater candidness of the participants' responses, the survey was confidential and the answers anonymous. Participants were asked—in a series of broad, open-ended questions—to identify and address the critical issues facing organized medicine and physicians through and beyond the year 2000.

As is to be expected in a survey involving a profession that has more than 600,000 members, the case with physicians, the responses reflect varying points of view and disagreement among them as well as agreement and sets of similar responses. Overall, their responses reflect a widespread and deep concern about the quality of healthcare and the structure of healthcare providers and delivery systems. The survey questions are listed in Appendix A as well as being presented in this chapter, each here with a discussion of participant responses.

Presentation of Responses

For two years I traveled and telephoned around the country, talking with individuals and groups, encouraging and prompting their responses and opinions, and recording what they said as efficiently as I could. In some cases they mailed their comments back to me. The transcriptions of their responses are voluminous. Instead of presenting them all here, I have distilled them, choosing quotes most

Survey and Responses

representative of many similar comments. Apart from quotes, this chapter's bulleted points and/or discussion derive from their responses and their attitudes as expressed (and then reviewed) in those raw responses. In some cases, my questions drew less response than I anticipated which may or may not reflect a lack of interest in the subject on their part.

Survey Question 1

What external forces are bringing about changes with Managed Care Organizations (MCOs)?

Respondents differentiated MCOs on the basis of quality, patient satisfaction, cost, improvements in explicit health outcomes; objective measures, benchmarks, and accreditation and evaluations (Health Employer Data and Information Set (HEDIS), National Committee for Quality Assurance (NCQA), Joint Commission on the Accreditation of Healthcare Organizations (JCAHO).

They identified these main forces:
- Increased competition
- Payer demands for higher levels of service at lower costs and better health outcomes
- Demographic shifts
- Sicker populations
- Risk adjustments
- Need to reduce days lost to illness
- Disease management programs

Survey Question 2

What are the internal pressures for changes in MCOs?
- Achieve a lower cost structure.
- Integrate services.
- Improve information management capabilities.
- Create data systems for a competitive and marketing edge. (Question: For what purpose?)
- Reduce budgets.
- Squeeze out costs.
- Improve healthcare delivery systems.

- Realign people and professional skills.
- Change routine activities of internal service units.
- Don't accept sick patients.

Survey Question 3

What are the major challenges in managing or leading physicians in MCOs and hospitals today?

"Business," said a pulmonary specialist who had made the transition from clinic to executive suite. He suggested that the major challenge in leading physicians is for physicians to develop organizational and business skills so that they can understand how healthcare delivery is being transformed and organized.

> *It is really moving the physician away from the model of 'I'm my own CEO,' to 'I'm a key member of the team that will be involved in a very focused way in changing healthcare delivery.' Also, it has always intrigued me that, generally, organizations have some of the brightest thinkers and the most effective operational people toward the top, then down through the organization are the worker bees. In medicine and healthcare, you have something very different.*

The problem stands regardless of disagreement among healthcare industry players: MCOs cannot manage medical cost.

Survey Question 4

What are the most critical challenges facing organized medicine in the next 3-5 years?

Is medicine business or patient care? Physicians are asking questions and their questions are unsettling, formidable. A pediatrician put his concerns before a group of peers:

> *Change is being forced by the economic demands of society. How are we going to maintain quality in patient care in the face of this? Most of us went into medicine to provide good services, to improve and maintain the health of the patients we serve. Most physicians are loath to see the quality suffer due to economic constraints. We have no track record showing that the changes occurring are going to make a difference. We now have these huge physician organizations, but there is no track record that the changes will improve anything in the next 5 to 10 years.*

Survey and Responses

> *The questions are: what will it improve, will our outcomes get better, will it drive cost out of the system, etc.? From a business standpoint it may be very good, coming in and buying hospitals, choosing which ones are going to close, but is that always good for the patients in the areas being served? The challenge to the physician is, how are we going to be relevant in this changing environment and still maintain the most critical dynamic, which is providing healthcare?*

The discussion among the physicians was energetic, revealing alternating feelings of discouragement and encouragement. When anger was evident, it centered on money:

> ***Why is it that when we are together these days, we don't seem to talk about medicine anymore. All we talk about is money! The cost and reimbursement issues always come up first.***

Payment and profit. The financial challenges are formidable and fear and resistance are common. Physicians are afraid to take risks and afraid of government interference, and they resist capitated payment and assuming risk. The method of payment is an ever-present concern. How much effect, they wonder, will attempts to balance the budget have on Medicare and Medicaid?

HMOs. The influx of HMO and private pay has and is eroding the patient/physician relationship that has basic to healthcare for a long time. Any relationship between a patient and a physician can be severed quickly by a simple change on the insurance company's part. Because the price of medical care is so high, most people can't go to a physician outside of the system dictated by their insurance company.

Lawsuits. Lawsuits, often trivial and usually won by physicians, also ruptures trust between patient and physician while consuming, wasting inordinate amounts of time.

Hospitals. Do we have too many hospitals? Hospitals are giving way to mobile practices because doctors may be on many medical staffs at once. To be part of several medical staffs' compounds insurance and assurance issues. Physicians want insurance, and also assurance of employment, begging the question of whether it may be better to combine medical staffs in healthcare, eliminating the rush to security in an effort to protect income flow. Is there any reason why hospitals cannot get into the insurance business and provide employment assurance at the same time? *Yes.* Hospitals manage less efficiently than do physicians and MCOs.

Johns Hopkins Hospital in Baltimore works with 4,000 payers—private, public, and governmental—only 992 of which have more than ten patients in the system annually. The administrative challenge is never-ending. With 4,000 payers, there are 4,000 paper and/or electronic systems to meet and satisfy. The possibility of error is immense. This system remains a world-class operation because of its ability to minimize error and ensure satisfaction. Smaller hospitals may not have 4,000 payers; nevertheless, they face the challenge of potential administrative nightmares, and so the question: why not a single payer system? I'm aware of the vigorous debate around this issue; I'm not aware of real dialogue.

Who in your healthcare system decides who gets what care and when? Since rationing and prioritizing care now happens daily, a person on medical assistance is not likely to get the same level of care as a bank president in most communities. If that happens today, and if healthcare is totally regionalized in 2010, which will care for the uninsured, the indigent, the forgotten? A physician nearing retirement reflected on what he anticipated in the future:

I would like to see a more unified voice and a commitment among physicians. This will take more time than most of us want to give. I think the younger physicians among us know the value of teamwork and common goals. We need to get physicians to join together with common goals and common missions. We should deliver care to everyone. We guarantee education through high school, why not healthcare? Eliminate waste in the system. Ninety percent of medical resources are often allocated during the last six months of life. This is an ethical dilemma.

Decision-making. The tyranny of the committee as a problem solver is another challenge. Hospitals and large clinics have far too many committees, which generate more committees, when a handful of core committees would be better. Most professionals dislike committees because they move at the speed of dark, aim at nothing, and hit it. Of all the physician leaders I've observed conducting meetings, only a handful knew how to manage both content and process. The rest of them needed a crash course on how to conduct productive meetings..

Regulations. In some states, the cost of medical education through residency is at or near $800,000 per student. There should be some

Survey and Responses

state or federal legislation allowing equal sharing of educational expense. The challenge for the general public and elected representatives is how to maintain quality in the face of staggering costs and reduced government support.

Customer service. A physician specializing in service to women surprised herself by speaking up. She wrote:

> *I'm surprised that I'm even thinking about marketing as a healthcare provider. I have become aware that we must market ourselves better, by becoming more customer-oriented. We have to delight patients with our care. We have to reach that level of expertise. I can't believe I just said that. For years I thought only about being a good physician; now I have to think about marketing myself first and being a physician second. There's something both crazy and right about that picture.*

Nurses and physicians.

A long-standing interpersonal issue in clinics, nursing homes, and hospitals is a distrust between nurses and physicians, usually about control and ownership. Like the elephant in the boardroom, everyone pretends it's not there. Distrust has been and will continue to be an issue until people find courage to address the concerns in the spirit of good will and not in the spirit of dominance.

New models of reimbursement.

The biggest challenge is determining how to deliver high or better quality care in an environment where resources to pay for that care seem to be stalled or shrinking. Provider organizations are being asked to bear more of the financial risk associated with care. Physicians, hospitals, and provider organizations together need to establish new care delivery models, and new fair reimbursement models within provider organizations that motivate people appropriately. Healthcare organizations need to find incentives to deliver superior performance in terms of efficiency, clinical quality, and service quality. Motivating people to change is a major management challenge.

Wall Street.

Walk into any doctor's lounge and hear conversation that is wide-ranging, often somber, containing references to money and the stock

Unraveling and Re-Birth

market. Here's a paraphrase of a common conversation I've heard among physicians:

> *A: Wall Street runs the medical field, for profit. Patient care will suffer greatly. I find that a great challenge. We're facing a rebellion. The cost of medicine is a universal problem. Socialized medicine also has failed.*
>
> *B: Medicine has become a business and business hurts patients. Business is for profit, which mostly is detrimental to patients. Business cares about the bottom line, not about patients. Our descent into the business mode must be modified to protect the welfare of patients. Tossing birthing mothers out of the hospital after one day, for example, and telling old people to go home, that nothing more can be done. These are business, not medical decisions.*

The conversation moves beyond Wall Street into more personal and related issues:

> *There are more than 75,000 of us here in California and more than 575,000 in the country. I think there are too many physicians and surgeons. We're going to have physicians getting into multi-level businesses to make ends meet.*

Employment security.

A firm declaration made in a physician's locker room was:

> *The time of job insecurity is here. I have a colleague who, with his wife, is selling Amway today. He thinks his future is dim in doctoring. We bought some of his products to get them started. He wanted us to become distributors, but we declined. He's all pumped about it. I wish he was as pumped up about being a physician.*

Quality control.

As the industry faces new kinds of constraints, quality control has become an important issue. Medical directors in long-term care are quick to point out that the nursing home industry is more highly regulated than the nuclear industry. Alternative medical practices are competing for medical dollars and many of them—chiropractic care and acupuncture, for example—haven't been proved "scientifically" to be quality care. Aromatherapy held in low regard in this country, is well regarded and widespread in England, Germany, and France and

Survey and Responses

even covered by some healthcare insurance. A respected national leader in internal medicine and geriatrics is concerned about new practices to deal with vulnerable people:

> *The most critical challenge is addressing the issue of incorporating high tech medicine and the medical model of care of the chronically ill. We need to analyze the effect of the overall model on the health of people and the quality of life. We assume that if it is high tech, it's better, but it has never been analyzed. The more medically involved and high tech, the more expensive, but we don't necessarily know if it is best for the patients' quality of life, especially if they are chronically ill.*

Generalists vs. specialists.

What will it take to call a truce between generalists and specialists? Continuing rapid increase in knowledge supports sub specializations, while managed care organizations and political pressures support generalists. Is healthcare better off because of the long-standing problems between generalists and specialists? It's amazing how poorly we deal with this problem, and it's more than a money issue.

A few years ago I was invited by the senior physician in a full-service clinic to discuss ways to improve communication among physicians. He reported that it was impossible for him to get the physicians in the same room to talk about how to improve the ways they dealt with each other: "They will talk with me, but they won't talk to each other." I asked what it was about him that encouraged communication with the physicians. He said, "I hired most of them. I'm the oldest in the group and I'm board certified as a specialist and in family practice. I'm a bit odd, I guess."

After I outlined a process that included confidential individual interviews, followed by a report on the issues and a discussion about options for individual and group development, he accepted the outline and said he would share it with all the partners. Later he said that he couldn't assemble the group to discuss the process because of their hostility toward the idea of discussing anything with people outside their discipline.

Declines in care? Patients today probably haven't had a serious decline in healthcare; it is possible for them if their access to healthcare is limited. A primary care physician wondered, "Most who have been in medicine for 10 years or more feel physicians and patients are less free to make choices about therapy and even the site of the therapy. Another physician said:

> *We are experiencing less access to patients, reduced fee schedules with resulting decreased income, while overhead continues to increase, and there are more prescribing restrictions through the use of formularies. This is one of the most disturbing developments in practicing medicine, with pharmaceutical companies more to be blamed than benefits people or providers.*

Organized medicine? A thoughtful ER physician in a focus group said:

> *Organized medicine is an oxymoron; medicine is not organized. Probably the most critical challenge is how to take a cottage industry, where there has been strong autonomy, and make it perform as a system. How do we take disparate and often competing interests, be they financing of care or the delivery of care from a hospital or physician-based source, and have it work as an organized, cohesive whole? That's the most critical challenge.*
>
> *The first challenge is to define how we use scarce resources in healthcare delivery. Today, with the age wave passing through the population, as well as the increasing contribution of health care to the GNP, we have to begin, if not to ration care, at least to rationalize care. That is a key issue. Second, provide access to the population. Third, be involved in the promotion of health. Fourth, I would look at consumer movement in healthcare as a key, so that the concept of informed decision-making makes patients partners in health care. Fifth, application of new and unproved technologies and how to introduce new, expensive technologies, and address the envelope on therapies at a time of constrained resources. Sixth, of course, is financial consideration for high quality care and gain-sharing. And probably the last one is how do you translate advances in basic biomedical research? I mean very potent advances in molecular biology and DNA where we're going to be able to identify problems at an earlier stage.*
>
> *Also, there's the ethical question of how to use these tools in the care of patients. But those are mighty challenges. You notice I didn't even get into the issues of for-profit healthcare versus not, or any of the mere, almost technical, models needed to deliver high quality, cost effective care.*

Survey and Responses

Another physician, part of a large healthcare delivery organization, saw humor in the notion of organized medicine:

> *Medicine is not organized, because no one knows how to organize it. Employers have driven the move to HMOs, which has tripled the amount of paperwork and increased the amount of support personnel needed to run a medical practice. In response, doctors seem to be assuming primacy of the doctor/patient relationship, cutting out the third party intermediaries who have done nothing more than remove the dollars from the healthcare system. The removal of dollars has led to physicians taking a pay cut.*

A colleague in the same focus group responsible for resident education ticked his points off on his fingers:

> *Physicians need to learn how to survive, how to work with the system and with management. Sometimes people don't want a doctor who is too good at management. It is important to try to maintain physicians' autonomy in much of the decision-making. We will have to maintain adequate reimbursement for physicians. And then there are also problems of integration.*
>
> *The Integration issues are: With whom do you integrate and how do you integrate? Physicians don't know with whom to align, how to align, and to what degree. Significant changes in practice strategies, trying to balance between efficiency and quality care. Many doctors are facing a significant reduction in economic status. The whole concept of care is tied up with how much doctors care about being doctors. A major challenge is to recapture the love of being a physician, what it means for patients and physicians themselves.*

A pulmonary specialist joined the spirited conversation with the admission that his thinking about systems and structures was a new experience for him and one that did not bring much pleasure:

> *Physicians are being challenged to figure out what organizational structure makes the most sense for them in their practice. What corporate structure is best for physicians in their practices? Physicians have to manage their practices much more closely than in the past. Patients have a much higher expectation about service. Physicians have to be much more critical about what is necessary to provide to make certain value is added to the patient's care. Insurance companies, the public and other physicians today are scrutinizing doctors' performance much more. Physicians have to*

Unraveling and Re-Birth

be accountable, not only for their ethical conduct, but for the quality and efficiency with which they practice.

Head-nodding assent among members of our focus groups supported the idea that physicians need to directly influence the decisions made by insurance companies, HMOs, and managed care. Physicians want to maintain quality of care outcomes for patients without over-utilizing resources. Resources are dwindling and physicians don't have any way to expand them through a policy standpoint. Insurance companies decide how money is spent, and doctors have to operate within those parameters. Example, sending mothers home within 24 hours of delivery.

Another concern stated repeatedly was:

I admit it frankly, I hate paperwork. The amount of paperwork a doctor has to do is obscene. Doctors are forced to enlarge their staffs without recompense just to handle the administrative part of the practice. And I dislike the whole concept of time management. We are expected to see 24 to 35 patients a day, and this gives us very little time to educate patients. We work harder and take home less pay. Now ask me how I really feel!

A medical society task force charged with finding new career paths in medical practice took on the added challenge of non-medical career pathways in healthcare. They began with the subject of job security:

Another challenge we've had to face for the first time in this century is just staying in practice. Being a physician used to be a secure field, now, for the first time, a doctor can fail. Some simply cannot stay in business. For example, a doctor in Nisswa, Minnesota had an independent practice. The HMOs wouldn't accept his bills and simply put him out of business. This, in essence, is saying that a doctor must be tied to an HMO to stay in business; they can no longer be independent.

Another person offered:

Doctors are arbitrarily losing their jobs because they become redundant in a merger. And young doctors and medical students are told that they may not find a job once they finish their training. This discourages many from taking on huge education loans for fear they won't be able to use their training as a profession. The public needs to know how tenuous we are in this position.

Survey and Responses

Another:

> With the changing role of physicians, maintaining professionalism is a major challenge. It's troubling that physicians are losing track of what it means to have a career. Physicians as employees have less regard for their personal/professional Curriculum Vitae accomplishments and have lost a sense of purpose, of belonging to a larger community. The landscape of medicine is changing: delivery of care, reimbursement for services, and the changing make-up of those who are entering medical school. Fee for service is dead unless a single payer plan other than Medicare is implemented.

Needed shifts in focus. The doctors' commentary reflects the need for some major shifts in our thinking and focus. The following list outlines some:

FROM	TO
Rapid change	Corporate groups, partnerships
Last quarter bottom line	Regional/national share
Cost control	Quality control, innovation, service
Small innovations	Fundamental change
New technology as cost	New technology as necessity
Focus on task	Focus on process
Status quo	Rapid change

The status quo holds a place of honor, respect, and safety in most organizations and has many proponents. Living organizations are in constant tension and, now, flux. Rules and restructuring arise from a need to control; after control is achieved, rules and structure may change again. In *Images of Organization*, Garth Morgan outlines the dynamic tension in organizations.

Innovate	vs.	Avoid mistakes
Think long-term	vs.	Deliver results now
Cut costs	vs.	Increase morale
Reduce staff	vs.	.Improve teamwork

Be flexible	vs.	Respect rules
Collaborate	vs.	Compete
Decentralize	vs.	Retain control
Specialize	vs.	Be opportunistic
Low costs	vs.	High quality

Innovate vs. Avoid mistakes, *e.g.*—In an organization that began small and is now a Fortune 500 giant, the founder instituted a program that announced and rewarded the Mistake of the Month. "Now we know what not to do," he said about mistakes. IBM had a great start.

Think long term vs. Deliver results now, *e.g.*—Currently healthcare is built on the illness model: I'm sick; make me better now. The new model is the wellness model: I want to be well for a long time; what must I do?

Cut costs vs. Increase morale, *e.g.*—Is this the message: 'Do more with less and feel good about it. We're going to cut your staff in half, give you more work and expect you to thank us for the privilege. When you're weary and at the end of your wisdom, be sure to remain positive and encouraged, and to uplift your co-workers. We're not asking for the impossible, just what's realistic.'

Reduce staff vs. Improve teamwork, *e.g.*—The push is on: 'Reduce more staff? Cut out half of the team? Yes. We know you're up to this. You've done great things before so just add this to your list of accomplishments. You're innovative and a great motivator, so let us know how you are doing so we can model this in other parts of the organization. Carry on.'

Be flexible vs. Respect rules, *e.g.*—There are wrong and right ways to do things around here. The customer must be our number one concern. So be flexible with the customer and remember that we can't have chaos. The customer has rules. We have rules. Sometimes the rules are in conflict. Serve the rules and the customer. Thank you.

Collaborate vs. Compete, *e.g.*—Work together, cooperate, and remember that we want a competitive edge. I will give you a little help on this one with a new way of thinking: The best way to compete is to cooperate.

Decentralize vs. Retain control, *e.g.*—We are in charge of this organization and we want to empower you to be in charge as well. The more people we have taking charge the more controls we will have in

Survey and Responses

the organization. We need this tension to survive and thrive. We have many units in this organization, too many for a few of us to manage. We want you to manage your unit and remember who is in control. It's simple.

Specialize vs. Be opportunistic, *e.g.*—Create a niche. Be a specialist. New opportunities will crop up every day so take advantage of them. You will need to be a generalist to see the new stuff so put on your wide-angle lenses and look through them with the eyes of the specialist.

Low costs vs. High quality, *e.g.*—We must buy what we need at the price of the Hyundai; at present our product is a Rolls Royce. Buy low. Sell high. You know the trick. Buy the best below wholesale and mark it up for high-end retail. Talk to every vendor that produces the best stuff. Do what you need to do to make money. Appearance must match reality. Everything must have quality stamped on.

Survey Question 5

What are physicians ill-equipped to do today? In the next 3 to 5 years?

Management. A surgeon with more than 35 years of experience responded with energy:

> *I believe that when you ask physicians, as I often do, if physicians lead the future of health care delivery, they say, 'Of course.' Take back the night, right? But the issue is that physicians have no management expertise, no capital, no ability to work in an organization, and basically are unwilling to sublimate their own personal interests for those of an organization. They tend to be driven, sadly, by financial security and that can get in the way of the best public policies for social issues. Think of the public health model in Western Europe. We haven't been anywhere. Our medical schools still teach students. Our hospitals don't train interns and residents—they're expected to master these areas on their own after training. And we don't teach the appropriate outcomes for search measures or resource utilization measures.*

A part-time pathologist/full-time vice president of medical affairs said:

> *What you do as a medical leader in practice and as a medical leader in administration are different. In practice everything is hierarchical. If you're in the ER and a patient comes in with a trauma, there's no question about what happens—you give the*

orders and people respond to the orders. In administration you sit around a table with 5-12 other people who also have opinions about what should be happening and it's a very different role. You have to use different skills, much more collaboration and consensus building. And remember that achieving consensus could also mean that no decision is made. I don't think we are training or equipping physicians to think in those terms. There would be benefits to teaching in medical school curriculum an awareness of social economics, consensus building, and collaboration.

Another physician observed:

Physicians who have moved into administrative leadership roles seem to come out of primary care, internal medicine, and pediatrics. Part of the reason that pediatrics is a source, for example, is that there you deal with more than the child; you deal with family, school, coach, and so on. So, you need to be collaborative. You can't just tear off a prescription and hand it to them. There may be a set of skills that you develop that makes the transition from practice to administration easier. I don't think it would be too difficult to incorporate some of those skills in medical schools, internship, and residency. Today's physicians are ill equipped to make this transition from specialists to primary care. The transition may come as a shock to those who have become used to a high lifestyle.

The leadership of physicians in medical administration may well require intentional leadership or MBA training and education at graduate school level before one can be employed in the pivotal positions of physician executives. The dilemma will continue to confront medical educators as well as those who are attracted to medicine and not management. A further comment:

Generally physicians have no business training, so they don't know how to run a business well. There's no business training in medical schools. An answer for that may be for integrated healthcare systems to employ physicians, or to take over the management responsibilities for their practices. That may create paranoia among physicians. Physicians may need private organizations to train them in the business aspects of running a medical practice. Physicians who are in administration and have stopped practicing medicine are known as suits. Usually it has more impact if the physician executive combines administrative

Survey and Responses

> *work with clinical practice and wears both suit and white jacket every week.*

Cost-effective medicine. The public and public policy makers will always want cost-effective healthcare. We need to continue establishing guidelines. Are national standardized guidelines and outcome measurements the answer? Is the United States too regionalized to support national standards of healthcare to ensure cost-effective medicine? Is cost-effectiveness possible when there is so much regional competition for patients? Could there be, for example, a sharing of epidemiologists and statisticians among regions to help hospitals hone the studies that they do?

Managed care. A cancer specialist who began his practice as a general surgeon has experienced considerable frustration with healthcare systems and is aware that there must be a lot of catching up and catching on before he and his colleagues are in a new medical comfort zone. He writes:

> *Most physicians don't understand what managed care is starting to do as far as practice guidelines, formulary guidelines, performance improvement measures, and overall report cards for physicians. They are angry and frustrated about it. There needs to be a huge amount of education for physicians about how we can look at that in a positive way. It might be a good thing in the long run. Physicians need to be convinced that by using these guidelines we're going to have better quality for our patients, and they're not convinced of that yet. We not only need to buy into it, we need to be part of the development.*

Keeping up with knowledge explosion. A primary care physician speaks for many of her colleagues.

> *Physicians are ill equipped to deal with the explosion of medical knowledge. A primary care physician is supposed to know everything. We're ill equipped to deal with the managed care system. Performance standards say that we're supposed to turn over patients rapidly. Our medical students are being taught to ignore the importance of the medical history because of the time factor.*

Historically, patients expected physicians to know everything about everything. Now, for less than the price of a steel-belted radial tire, a consumer can purchase a CD that contains more information than a person will retain from medical education. Potentially, consumers can be as well informed as any physician on any medical subject; in most cases consumers are not prepared to integrate the data in order to make an accurate diagnosis.

Business decisions, patient care, death. A continuing frustration for many physicians is that medical decisions now are equated with business decisions while physicians are not equipped to insist on the kind of care they want for their patients. It has become a business transaction in which care often is determined on the basis of cost, and when cost becomes the final argument, care is likely to lose.

Given the considerable media exposure to Dr. Kevorkian and physician-assisted suicide, many physicians feel ill equipped to deal with death. Ethical issues surrounding life's end stages are not discussed clearly and forthrightly in medical school, nor are the difference between morality and ethics. Informed by cultural mores, morality may focus on what we can get away with, while ethics is prescriptive and oriented to professional behavior. As a philosophical subject or a decision-making aid, ethics transcends cultural codes of conduct. What is moral in Iraq, for instance, may be penalized in Illinois; what one can get away with in Illinois may be penalized severely in Iraq. Many physicians are not prepared to deal with these aspects of another person's life.

Decision-making. Often physicians find decision-making within large healthcare systems distasteful because they see their decisions subsequently slip down a rabbit hole. Physicians are trained to be decisive and see the results of their decision-making. Consuming time to deal with divergent points of view and trying to build consensus can be repugnant to them. When dealing with issues not related to patient care, they are equally sensitive. A senior partner in a clinic serving a community of 75,000 writes:

> *Physicians need to learn new skills, disciplines, and the ability to position our practices to meet the challenges successfully of an evolving marketplace. One problem is dealing with huge personnel problems that a physician may perceive as minor. Physicians in our clinic tend to dismiss petty stuff quickly, but what is a nosebleed to one may be life threatening to another. I have sought administrative help to solve these issues.*

Survey and Responses

Given the dramatic increase of mergers and acquisitions in healthcare, a physician executive was quick to point out a problem area:

> *A primary issue for physicians is that they are poorly equipped to deal with change or manage change. Traditional training takes an enormous amount of time, and the concepts of being a physician are rooted so early in one's career that changing direction quickly is hard.*
>
> *Many medical schools today, including the Baylor College of Medicine, have introduced into the curriculum courses that might be entitled "The Patient, Physician and Society." As part of that and similar courses, physicians are being trained in issues of the economics of medicine, and they're being trained more extensively in interpersonal relationships and how to interact with people in many different areas besides just the patient. They're being trained more extensively than previously about a number of biomedical ethical issues that are very important because in a capitated environment they're paid a flat sum for a given person, ill or not. The goal of capitation is to reduce costs, but there's an unfortunate side effect not to provide all the care that should be provided. So physicians must hold the highest ethical values in order to treat patients while withstanding external forces that might keep them from providing appropriate treatment.*

Survey Question 6

What are the major challenges faced by physicians today? In the next 3 to 5 years?

Four Issues. A physician executive in a large healthcare delivery system answered at length, finding four principal issues. He wrote:

> *This is something we have asked physicians in polls, focus groups, and other approaches. The first challenge is how can we balance autonomy and critical decision making with the consistency of a product? Second, how can we deal with financial security and an established lifestyle, when medical resources are going to be diminished, which is the case most often for specialists? Third, how can we overcome our own cultural issues when we believe that patients and others should respect our very difficult task of taking care of patients, while increasingly people view us as assembly line workers? Fourth, what is the role of physician*

practice management companies' consolidation and organization within the practice of medicine?

Autonomy. Another respondent spoke to the issue of independence:

> There's a tremendous sense of loss of autonomy. Part of the appeal of medicine has always been the doctor-patient relationship, which is very one-on-one. More and more there is a sense of interference. Physicians are not empowered to deal with their patients the same way as in the past. It's disturbing to physicians that there is a set time for discharging patients, not looking at the parameters: the age of the patient, will they be able to function out of the hospital, is there a support system out there for them. The day of solo practice is becoming increasingly more difficult to maintain. Even if you have an office, you'll need to be linked to other physicians. Today's physicians feel that they have no worth. Historically, they were revered. Society has become cynical of physicians the same way they are cynical of politicians. That is a huge shock for doctors who are dedicated to their practices.

Incentives. Why would any healthcare system create incentives for a physician not to treat a patient? A physician in private practice and on the faculty of a medical school criticized the capitation reimbursement system:

> I think that I've always felt ethical physicians do what is right for patients regardless of which way the incentives are aligned. And I think most physicians, before we were in a capitated environment, did not over-treat patients and did not order tests simply to run up the bill. If there were some people then who abused that system, I can assure you they will be the same people who will abuse any other system regardless of how the incentives are arranged. But an ethical physician should do and does do what is correct for patients regardless of how incentives happen to be aligned.

A colleague in the same focus group who is responsible for resident education said:

> Physicians need to learn how to survive, learn how to work with the system and with management. Sometimes people don't want a doctor who is too good at management. It is important to try to maintain physician's autonomy in much of the decision-making. We will have to maintain adequate reimbursement for physicians. And then there are also problems of integration.

Survey and Responses

Integration issues: with whom do you integrate and how? Physicians don't know with whom to align, how to align, and to what degree. [These are] significant changes in practice strategies, trying to balance between efficiency and quality care. Many doctors are facing a significant reduction in economic status. The whole notion of care is tied up with how much doctors care about being doctors. A major challenge is to recapture the love of being a physician, what it means for the patients and for the physicians themselves.

Information. We have to remember to connect the dots. Information out of context is just an unconnected dot. A diagnosis out of context is another dot. I heard two surgeons who were relaxing during a coffee break at a continuing medical education workshop. Their free-flowing conversation was portentous as they talked about the "hip in 232."

"Is that hip connected to anything?" I interrupted.
"Of course, are you joking?"
"I'm not a physician. Tell me, what's the hip connected to?"
"Now you're being silly."
"Perhaps. Is that hip somehow connected to a face?" I insisted.
"Sure, it belongs to a woman."
"Then that face belongs to a person, right?"
"Right. Where's this going?"
"Does that person have a name?"
"Of course."
"What is her name?"
No answer.
"You might be talking about my wife, doctors, and I assure you, she's more than just a hip."

A diagnosis made out of context is an isolated dot. Without a clear frame of reference, it is meaningless. "We have entered a new Middle Ages," writes Michael Ventura, "a time of plagues, famines, violence, extreme class disparity, and religious fanaticism, and also, as in the late Middle Ages, a time of profound discovery and change. A time when it is terribly important, and often dangerous, to preserve values and knowledge, to stand up for visions that most of this crazed world can't comprehend or tolerate."

A physician who knows how to connect the dots, and knows that computers cannot solve our need for information or connect our human dots said:

A physician needs to be able to deal with the changing face of medicine and the technologies that are available, staying up to date on the latest medical information regarding new diseases and new procedures. The population is getting older. The issues facing the majority of patients are also changing.

Another person said:

Physicians are challenged to maintain academic research. Maintaining academic research and developing activities is key to the continuation of preeminent medicine being practiced in the United States.

Another:

Regulatory changes clearly are impacting medicine and there are caps on which they work for. For example, in the state of Minnesota over half of all physicians work for corporations and within the structure of a business. This is a big change from 20 years ago when physicians ran their own offices. Now there are regulations and policies that govern the physician that are being managed by the gatekeeper. For example, to see a specialist, a patient must go through the HMO to get a referral.

To connect the dots in the midst of all such pressures, doctors might reconsider their basic work values. The work dimensions of most professional healthcare providers are often referred to as value dimensions. In their model based on their research on the world of work, Dawis and Lofquist of the University of Minnesota have identified six value dimensions of work:

Value	Need Scale	Importance Statement from the Minnesota Importance Questionnaire
Achievement	1 Ability utilization	I could do something that makes use of my abilities
	2 Achievement	The job could give me a feeling of accomplishment
Comfort	3 Activity	I could be busy all the time
	4 Independence	I could work alone on the job
	5 Variety	I could do something different every day
	6 Compensation	My pay would compare well with that of other workers
	7 Security	Provide steady employment
	8 Working conditions	Good working conditions

Survey and Responses

Status	9 Advancement	The job would provide an opportunity for advancement
	10 Recognition	I could get recognition for the work I do
	11 Authority	I could tell people what to do
	12 Social status	I could be somebody in the community
Altruism	13 Co-workers	Co-workers easy to make friends with
	14 Moral Values	Work without feeling it is morally wrong
	15 Social service	Do things for other people
Safety	16 Policies and Practices	Policies administered fairly
	17 Supervision: human relations	Supervisor backs me up
	18 Supervision: technical	Adequate training provided
Autonomy	19 Creativity	Could try out my ideas
	20 Responsibility	Make decisions on my own

Survey Question 7

What are the major challenges faced by hospitals today? In the next 3-5 years?

Fading epicenter. A hospital administrator in a focus group had been thinking about this question:

> *The major challenges faced by hospitals, I think, are three. One is to get rid of their Oedipus complex. Obviously, I say that with some cynicism, but I think the hospitals no longer will be viewed as the center of the universe. They are important components in the delivery of health care, but increasingly they have to engage their medical staffs in the effective delivery of care. The days of finding the low-hanging fruit of hospitals' improvement of financial performance are over. The food service is outsourced. The linen is being done in a consolidated laundry. All of that is taking place.*
>
> *Now, it's about optimizing the medical care process, that's the future. But I think part of it is to engage physicians as true partners. Interestingly, around here they're called key customers. I believe that physicians are partners, here to serve our customers. I have a little different read on it than others and I think, of course, one does have to treat physicians and their customers as customers if you're providing an array of services.*

> The second is how do hospitals take the huge capital they've amassed and basically reinvent themselves? Obviously, that's what systems like ours are doing and maybe systems like Partners.
>
> And the last is, who will lead the development of clinical integration? Will physicians lead it? Well, sadly, they have no capital, no organization. Will health plans lead it? Sadly, they don't have the staying power and they're not committed to the enterprise. So, I think the hospitals have to pull the financing and the physicians together with the capital they have and, really, I don't want to say lead it, but at least support it in a major way.

An executive vice president of medical affairs in a system with more than 20 hospitals commented on these changes facing hospitals:

> Hospitals will change significantly. I think hospitals no longer will be the epicenter of delivery. If we look at Medicare today, probably 40% to 50% of the healthcare dollars are going into hospitals or the associated ambulatory care environment. I think we'll see a redistribution of that income. So, first hospitals will have to become much more efficient in how and when they build services. Then I think we'll see less of an arms race, and more of a community-wide rationalization of services. So that will be one theme.
>
> I think the second theme will be that hospitals will have develop some of the service features of retail industries and operate from a service platform. It won't be good enough for hospitals to operate five days a week and treat patients as being fortunate just to be in that institution. This will involve all hospitals, both profit and not-for-profit because we are beginning to see a backlash against for-profit hospitals. When you look at some very large hospital holders, there is what appears to be a systematic misrepresentation of illness rather than more efficient management. We're going to have lots of internal reviews and benchmarking to achieve optimal performance. Hospitals will take talented people from industries other than healthcare that will become future leaders of hospitals. I think you'll see more physician executive leaders of hospitals.

Survey Question 8.

What specialties will disappear, change, or be assimilated in the next 3 to 5 years?

Survey and Responses

As expected, specialists and primary care physicians approached this question from their own occupational perspectives. There is no intellectual unanimity among physicians about the future of specialization. A specialist said:

> *I think that we will see the pendulum swing dramatically away from primary care to specialty care. When you look at models developed initially by Foundation Health Systems and at the Oxfords where there's been effective management, the change isn't in carving out disease, but in developing expertise in disease-state management. It's putting resources behind that complexly ill diabetic or the patient with congestive heart failure. If anything, specialties will be transformed again and I think we'll see the rise of a specialty of principal care doctor, as opposed to primary care doctor. For example, an endocrinologist/diabolist can probably do a better job with a complex diabetic patient than a generalist. We will have to integrate that care through extraordinary events in technology and information systems and bring those disparate silos of care together in a common consortium.*

A primary care perspective:

> *In general, I don't see much disappearing. But I think we'll see specialty development along functional lines. For example, in women's services there will be obstetrics/gynecology, naturally, but it may be with someone involved in nutritional health or an endocrinologist who's studying bone disease and treating skeletal fractures, and people dealing with breast disease and breast surgery. But most important, there will be a wellness focus.*

A cardiologist views the future of specialties from the standpoint of disease:

> *Care will develop around two areas. One is geographic, and the other might be disease organized around service lines. Look at the organization of heart services, for example, where we have cardiologists, cardiac surgeons, physiologists, people who are focused on lipid metabolism, on exercise and rehabilitation, who all work together as units as opposed to more traditional disciplines of cardiology, cardiac surgery.*

A medical affairs executive trained in internal medicine is concerned about integrating medical care before systems disintegrate:

Unraveling and Re-Birth

> *What we do is make it real on day-to-day operations. For example, integration today in heart services may mean sitting down and having a common approach to a patient with chest pain or TMI applied across the system. It may be looking at how we manage resources and why it's important for different levels of cost and different outcomes. But it's also how can we build market share at heart services. So, I'm not only speaking as a clinician on clinical care as a system; it's a marketing effort. How do we win this market, how do we get 40-45% market share if that's what we can do before the FTC starts looking at what we're up to. The important question is about integrated care, not about specialists or generalists. That's the business case that we have to make and we want physicians involved very much in the business case.*

An executive vice president of medical affairs in a public healthcare system and trained as a specialist writes:

> *They won't disappear, but numbers will diminish in some specialties by natural attrition. Some won't be needed any more. Some areas of primary care will be at risk. You may see a pediatrician overseeing four or five PAs and have cases referred rather than being the primary caregiver. Anesthesiology may all but disappear. There will be fewer obstetricians. Some specialty numbers will decrease but won't disappear. Cardiologists will decrease in number. The role of the primary doctor will be a case-manager role, managing advanced nurse practitioners and physician's assistants.*

A primary care physician is concerned about the increased load put on the family practitioner:

> *I don't think specialties will disappear, but specialists will, and there will be a trend towards primary care. I hope the primary care physicians will be prepared to handle the load and the level of expertise for specialty patients. We may regret the shift, patients may suffer lessening of quality care if primary care doctors are forced to perform some specialties without the level of expertise of specialists.*

A specialist writes about potentially redundant over-care.

> *There may be a difference between family practice and internal medicine. Both are considered primary care physicians, but merging the two is possible. It may be more cost-effective for patients who come to the hospital to be treated by doctors in the*

Survey and Responses

> *hospital rather than their primary care physicians. The role of critical care physicians is not clear; it might not be necessary for a critical care doctor, a cardiologist, and a primary care doctor all to care for the same patient.*

An East Coast specialist examines the future from the perspective of the public:

> *Specialists outnumber primary care physicians. Studies indicate that patients with certain conditions who are managed by specialists rather than primary care physicians do better and the costs are less. At some point we'll see the primary care "star" flatten out and descend. If we go down the capitation path, less costly workers will be substituted for higher cost workers. The public won't go for that. Medicine can't continue to be good and get better if we don't maintain specialties. There will always be a need for experts, specialists. There will be fewer people in the fields, but there will always be a need for them.*

A physician trained in internal medicine and now specializing in geriatrics looks at the continuum of care:

> *In contrast to the other specialties, geriatrics is one specialty that is gaining interest, and is, in fact, incredibly robust due to a rapidly aging population and an increased demand to meet their needs. Along with geriatrics is the area of senior housing, home care and assisted living facilities. The AMDA (American Medical Directors Association) is working to expand its membership base by embracing hospice home care and assisted living. Many of these organizations are taking on medical directors, even though by law they are not required, improving the quality of the organization with physician leadership.*

A surgeon with more than 30 years of experience is convinced that there will be more specialists in the future based on the explosion of new information, new diseases, and new technologies.

> *I don't believe that any specialty will disappear, because the specialty wouldn't exist if there wasn't a reason for its existence. I do think the change will be in how medicine is practiced. The numbers in certain specialties will decrease but not disappear. Quite the contrary, I believe new specialties will develop. As we begin to apply molecular biology and advances in gene medicine in the form of gene therapy to clinical problems, we'll see a*

> variety of physicians who are skilled both in molecular biology and in the transfer of that knowledge to clinical medicine.

A podiatrist writes:

> Most medical administrators are not concerned about this question, but about business. I think the momentum is to run medicine more and more as a business, and while we favor doing things efficiently and effectively, we have to remember that medicine is not, in a classic sense, a business. It is a profession and it's a profession because you're dealing with the people's health and people are individual. Although we have guidelines for various diseases and teaching how to treat patients most efficiently, there will always be variations on the theme.

Hospitals, for the most part, are independent silos and they need to re-invent themselves. The re-invention must include a seamless integration, a true continuum of care.

Survey Question 9

What changes will be necessary to make in practicing medicine in the next 3 to 5 years?

The future is scary for some, exciting for others, and uncertain for most, while it's an opportunity to create and innovate for all. We asked our contributors to reach into the future to imagine what lies ahead in establishment medicine, medical education, alternative medicines, the place of spirituality, and the focus of healthcare—patients.

Alternative medicine. A hematologist took an overview:

> We don't have any idea what's going to happen with alternative medicine. There is some alternative medicine that is helpful. Stress management, massage therapy, etc., may become incorporated into traditional medicine because patients will demand it. We will have to provide that to meet the needs of patients. Patients are going to demand more direction to their own education so they have more control over some of their life. If you're chronically ill, you have the right as a patient to know what's going on for making decisions. Informed consent. Patients are going to demand more control over their own destiny. I think medicine is going to have to respond to that in a variety of ways.

Survey and Responses

Physicians are aware of and skilled in alternative medicine to varying degrees; many haven't a feel for what's going to happen. Biofeedback stress management, massage therapy, chiropractic, herbal therapies (ayurvedic medicine), aromatherapy, music therapy, etc., are being used by many physicians and may be incorporated into allopathy because patients will demand it and will seek out physicians who offer it. Patients will demand more direction, more education, more understanding about their treatment, so they can be partners in their own healthcare. Chronically ill patients have the right to know what's involved in their medical future. The issue is informed consent and it's more common every day.

Complementary medicine. A pediatrician wrote:

Complementary medicine, like chiropractic care and holistic medicine have become more popular because it looks at the whole person. Traditional physicians have forgotten to treat the whole patient, as a member of a family, or of a community, and as a spiritual being.

Spirituality and health. A recent survey of over 200 doctors conducted at the annual American Academy of Family Physicians has found that an overwhelming 99% agree that spiritual beliefs can help patients heal. The survey found also that 80% of the doctors, men and women of all ages nationwide; believe that learning how to use relaxation or meditation techniques or both with patients should be part of formal medical training.

In a study of more than 1700 North Carolina adults aged 65 and over, Duke University researchers found that people who attend religious services at least once a week have healthier immune systems than those who don't: "It's the first study ever published in the medical literature that has found an association between religious activity and immune functioning," said Dr. Harold Hoenig, director of Duke's Center for the Study of Religion/Spirituality and Health. Chaplain David Carl, director of pastoral care and education at Carolinas Medical Center in Charlotte, said he's not surprised at the finding. "Our beliefs show up, right now, in our biology. We're all one. Our beliefs and our biologics are interconnected."

A medical director, concerned about the relevancy of physicians, spoke with firm conviction:

We will have to shift our focus for treating patients more to the outpatient setting. Hospitals are gearing down as far as what they do in an inpatient setting. In order to continue well economically, we have to be extremely efficient in outpatient care. Doctors have to make sure they continue to educate themselves or they will not stay up to date. In order to practice medicine, we have to be involved in other levels: the community, the government etc.

Working as both a physician and an administrator he addressed both administrative and education issues:

We need to become more sensitive to costs. It is more critical now than ever that we are not wasting money...Physicians have a responsibility to teach their patients, not just fix them. Yet, with the ever-increasing demand to see more and more patients, we have less time to do this. Educating patients is poorly reimbursed. However, better HMOs are now convinced that it is important to teach its patients to be healthy; this improves their bottom line. Prevention is better than treating a disease.

We need a system that runs smoothly; we have to pay attention to what people really want. We need a healthcare system that provides for everybody. Physicians will organize into larger groups and give up autonomy. Less personal and more anonymous. Physicians will use more technology to provide better care.

"It will be necessary to involve physicians in the decision-making process relative to insurance coverage. We need to make sure that the decision about coverage and care is not made solely by a clerk in an insurance office sitting behind a computer with a big medical book. Physicians must be involved.

But we need to look at the way we practice medicine—we need to set up guidelines on how to use the technology we have. For example, for the individual who is at the end of his life, the legal profession says that we need to use the most high-tech equipment and costly hospital stays, when it may not be what the patient really wants—but they are subjected to care. Different groups define quality of care differently: physician, legal, patient. This is a system-wide issue, a tough one to tackle.

We need to find the resources to continue to do research. We can't turn back the clock, and we must continue to learn—if our research is lost, medicine will be too.

Survey and Responses

Reasons for failure. In 1920, the average American baby could expect to live to only fifty-four years. Who, then, could have predicted that in 1990, average life expectancy would climb to seventy-five years, seventy-two for men and nearly seventy-nine for women? Who could have predicted AIDS in 1945? Who can predict what kind of institutions will be successful in 2010? We can better anticipate the future by examining the past and the present. We know why hospitals and medical practices fail. It is likely that our future successes will depend on how well we learn from our failures. The following figure identifies some patterns of our failures. See if these apply to the institutions you know.

Great Hospitals/Long-Term Care Facilities and Their Patterns of Failure

Unparalleled track record of success	Accumulation of abundant resources	Optimized Business System	Success confirms strategy
No gap between expectations and performance	A view that Resources will win out	Deeply Etched Recipes	Momentum is mistaken for leadership
Contentment with current performance	Resources Substitute for creativity	Vulnerability to new rules	Failure to "reinvent" leadership
Inability to escape the past		**Inability to invent the future**	

You might consider auditing your organization with related questions, such as these:
- If your organization is successful, to what do you attribute your success?
- If your organization is borderline, what needs to be addressed?
- If your organization is failing, find the land mines.
- What in your organization prevents people from searching for and finding systemic, root causes of failure?

  A radiologist responsible for physician and organizational development, when asked to summarize the conversation of a focus group, provided a full summary:

We are here to provide good healthcare for all. There will continue to be tough economic, moral, ethical, and legal issues. Can we keep a personal calling to medicine alive. How to care for people where you have and not be financially incentivized. Doing some procedures will cost us more money; it's a dilemma. Invent a new system which is outcome based. More women are entering the medical field. Many will be having children. We haven't thought about the impact on manpower with maternity leave. Alternative medicine will be huge in the future. The aging of the population will make demands on the system. The abandonment of the children in our society, they're uninsured. The gulf will become greater between children of well-off families and those from poor homes."

Drop-in medicine has the potential to hurt depending on quality control. Doctors should be compelled to continue their education and be re-certified. Someone will have to take control of physicians remaining competent. Doctors will continue to fight with systems and facilities. Payers will continue to try to get every single dollar they can out of the system. The government will have to be a part of the medical field. The government ought to go in full blast. It would take a long time to implement socialized medicine. We need to have Family-Centered Care. We have to understand the variables in the different cultures. Leaders might be better appointed rather than elected. It can be a popularity contest with elections. We are going to have an exceedingly large number of older people. New viruses will be appearing.

It became obvious that her note taking and presentation had been extensive and also internalized. She continued:

We have to recognize we can't just say what is good or bad in isolation. We need to look at the common good. Its ethical issues—issues of justice. Do we spend money on one bone marrow transplant or immunize 1000 kids with the same money? Tough questions. Cloning will have an unbelievable impact on medicine in the future. No telling the impact. Genetic splicing will also have impact.

Maybe a single payer will help smooth out bumps in the road. I expect that there will be a general move away from capitation toward more discounted fee for service with some new mechanism ultimately being developed to finance education, research, and care for the uninsured.

Survey and Responses

I began in this book by talking about the unraveling—some prefer to call it changing—of healthcare. Healthcare does not exist in a vacuum. Our society is held together by seen and unseen infrastructures. America, I believe, is built on and around at least seven major fault lines: ***economic, social, cultural, technological, ecological, political, military, educational and spiritual.*** The tension between societal good vs. individual utility stretches across them all.

If our economic life unravels with mounting public debt, trust funds in bankruptcy, unemployment, hyperinflation or debilitating deflation, and collapsing financial markets, the other fault lines will start to crack. If armed gangs rub our social fault lines raw, racial violence, extremist militias, and class feuds, we will be in continuous distress. If our cultural fault lines are monitored by governmental control in effect, we will suffer national decay.

If our technological fault lines shape life around machines served by people, we will lose our individual and national soul. If our ecologies are uncared for, we will consume contaminated water and food, and new diseases will constantly confront us. If our political life succumbs to a one-party superpower, we will have tax revolts, secession of states from the union, and re-defined borders. If our military is too weak or too strong, we may be overcome by terrorists or inflict mass destruction on the rest of the world and ourselves. This is the ultimate distress.

The cultural fault line here is elaborated by Josh Hammond's research on the "Stuff Americans are made of." Hammond defines seven cultural forces that shape us: *Insistence on choice, Pursuit of impossible dream, Obsession with big and more, Acceptance of mistakes, Urge to improvise, Fixation on what's new.*

So, what's at stake? Everything, including healthcare.

Soteria. The Greek word for salvation, *soteria,* means health. As a physician, you are encouraged to lead us into new realms of health. You are encouraged to teach us how to *see* those realms. We need to see a new world that is safe, healthy, productive, and loving. You are a helper, a healer, a teacher, and a leader. We need your gifts of intelligence, knowledge, caring, and hope.

A veteran pediatrician turned medical-executive answered question 9 from an operational point of view.

I think first physicians will have to change. Historically, some of the most sophisticated approaches have been taken in the former staff of group model HMOs, like Kaiser's, Group Health, and Harvard Community Health Plan. I think those physicians who've been in basically IPA or community based practice have to embrace many of those principles of groupness. Additionally, many of the former staff physicians have to embrace some of the principles of performance and, I will use that horrible word, efficiency. But I think at the end of the day it's not going to be about who can generate money and who can develop the productivity formulas, it's going to be that physicians need to be rewarded on five platforms, and the first of those is medical resource management.

The second is quality with measurable difference and outcomes. The third is patient satisfaction. But the other two that are key for physicians because of their collaborative nature are, four, building rewards for being a team player; and five, balancing those rewards with commitments to renew professionals, whether in teaching, clinical research, or just excellence in clinical care and community work. I think we'll see more groups coming together. We'll see medical partners grow. We'll see a great shakeout in this industry. We'll see physician-led organizations dominating the landscape. Physicians are allowing Wall Street to run medicine because physicians, I think, have tended to look near-term. We serve near-term problems; we're not looking ahead 10 or 20 years.

Integrated system or HMO? A neurologist writes:

Going back to the changes occurring, I suggest that the integrated health care system is the way to go, not the integrated delivery system. There are so many things occurring right now. Patients and people will start to demand things, no matter what employers' insurance companies say. The perfect example of that is the drive-through delivery, to which the grass-roots response was, "Enough! You just can't shove us out the door 24 hours after having a baby." Patients want choice, access, not to be treated as a bottom-line commodity. That will impact what happens in medicine. Also, people will become more demanding of community kinds of things."

Vertical integration. The vertical integration of healthcare delivery systems will continue. The development of integrated medical records will allow for rapid transfer of accurate medical information. Evidence-

Survey and Responses

based medicine will be the basis for many medical decisions. Physicians will need to focus on wellness care and preventive medicine.

A surprising point of view came from an anesthesiologist:

Going back to the changes occurring, I would no longer predict that the integrated delivery system is the way to go. HMO is the way to go. There are so many things occurring right now. Patients will demand things no matter what employers' insurance companies say. The perfect example of that was the drive-through delivery. The grass-roots response became: 'Enough, you can't just deliver have a baby and shove [mother and child] out the door in 24 hours.' It got to be a political issue. Patients want choice, they want access. They don't want to be treated as just a bottom-line commodity. That will impact what happens in medicine. People will become more demanding of community kinds of things, too. I think you're going to see a rise in health.

Medical Education. There is a debate among policy makers, government funding agencies, and medical education specialists that medical schools are producing more physicians than this country needs. It is estimated that we have too many medical schools by about one third. If one third of the schools were closed or merged, the quality of training and education would not be diminished. There would be very little faculty displacement since most of the instructors are engaged in a private or system practice and serve as adjunct to the medical school faculty. However, closing medical schools is a subject as politically volatile as closing military bases.

One survey respondent wrote:

Academic institutions traditionally have focused on delivery of state-of-the-art medical care at the cutting edge of knowledge and applying recent research advances to individual patients' care. In addition, academic medical centers traditionally are where people were trained, whether they were going into general practice or sub-specialization. The sub-specialists then would practice or join an academic medical school faculty where they participated in educating future physicians, did research, and cared for patients in their area of expertise.

Diminishing clinical income from attempts to control healthcare costs, particularly in managed care, means that income previously earned in academic centers from the surplus derived from clinical activities and put into the support of education research is lessening or non-existent. Thus, research support, particularly prior to funding by external organizations, must be sought from other difficult to obtain sources. So difficult, that research enterprise may cease to exist. In addition, income supporting people who teach part-time and full-time, will have to come from other sources."

Outpatient treatment. Physicians and hospital administrators are aware that we will have to shift our focus to treating patients as outpatients, and hospitals are gearing down their inpatient setting. In order to do well economically, physicians have to provide care extremely efficiently, keep their continuing education up to date and be involved in other levels of the community and government. The independent, autonomous physician is a dinosaur.

A general surgeon, comfortable with conversations about science, technology, and patient care gave thoughtful consideration to the question of changing practices in medicine.

I think future physicians, in the year 2000, 2010 and beyond, will have to be very firmly grounded in molecular biology and also computer literate, because now a lot of information is available instantly on the Internet and from sources other than just the traditional medical journals or textbooks. Moreover, I believe future physicians will need increasing competence in things like telemedicine, where they will do consultations at a distance. This may even be true of primary care physicians who may see a patient in the patient's home from their own home.

I think that physician executives will need the same competencies as a general physician, and they will need competencies in management, finance and business. A lot of today's physician executives moved into their position without those skills and acquired them on the job. Medical schools are beginning to recognize the need to incorporate these skills in the ordinary curriculum.

Survey Question 10

In the future, what new technical and non-technical competencies will physicians need to develop to continue to be effective?

Survey and Responses

Realizing that she had not been involved in a professional development experience for three years other than CME (Continuing Medical Education) courses provided at trade fairs, this OB-GYN with less than five years of experience said:

> *I think it's learning how to really respond to customer/patient needs, how to apply the scientific framework of medicine to the compassion and passionate care that is given, understanding when and how to involve all of the talented healthcare people in the care process. It's developing an appreciation of understanding the needs of patients along with a proactive approach to having patients become accountable for their health. What competencies won't be necessary in the future will be some of those that are just burdensome, the 'administrivia' that many physicians find themselves immersed in because they've no one else to do it.*

Respondents were asked to answer the same question for physician executives. A radiologist with an interest in systems development enjoyed talking about executive development. He knows the language and the process:

> *Physician Executive. That has intrigued me because I was actually recommending to a physician today that she spend some time in an executive MBA program. I think the physician executives need to learn many, many skills. There are broad business skills, management skills, negotiation skills, performance measurement, business planning, driving. We can go through a litany of business skills that physicians need as they become executives. Probably the key skill that we/they need is appreciating the business model and being responsive to that while also being responsive to their basic goals and clinical care delivery.*

On the other side of competency is incompetency. According to *Public Citizen*, a consumer health advocacy group in Washington, D.C., fewer than one third of incompetent doctors across the country have been prevented from practicing even temporarily by the state medical boards charged with monitoring them. To help patients identify problem physicians, *Public Citizen* has a state-by-state listing of questionable doctors in the United States.

Survey Question 11

What changes will be necessary to deal with external organizations such as the third- party payer?

Unraveling and Re-Birth

A 57-year-old podiatrist spoke with conviction and clarity:

We have to get data. Nobody has the systems to get data. I am very excited about the physician network that we're developing because I think it's going to forge a mechanism to do ambulatory as well as inpatient work. If you can go to a third party payer and say, 'This is how we're handling our diabetics, and these are the outcomes we're looking for, and this is how we're measuring it. We don't have much data now, but this is the system we've put in place.' I think they're going to perk up their ears, because I don't think people are doing that. That's my mission, because if we do that we will improve patient care. We're going to become less acute-care hospitals and we'll be seeing more chronic disease. We are going to have to learn how to manage diabetes, and coronary artery disease, congenital heart failure, asthma, etc., in a better way than we do now, in a less fragmented, smoother way. That's where the changes are going to have to come.

His tone became more serious when he spoke of contracts:

There needs to be more attention to outcome measures that are easily acquired. We've gone from fee-for-service where you're still giving decent rates, but you contract on an individual basis. The payers would come to each practice and say, 'This is the contract, sign if you want to work with us.' Now the contracts go through bigger organizations, where you have managed care organizations being the single signature for a group of physicians, or you have groups of physicians with some type of single-signature authority for their group. The insurance companies are coming directly to the physicians saying, 'Sign this individual contract with us.'

He expressed a strong concern for physicians negotiating with physicians:

Now we have spokespersons for groups of insurance companies negotiating contracts with managed care. Or we have larger groups of professional administrators assigned just to the task of managed care negotiations. If we could get a better level of trust with external organizations and more cooperation with them, it would work better. That takes a little give and take on both sides. Do external organizations such as insurance companies add value to patient care? More negotiation with docs by docs with third-party payers.

Survey and Responses

> *I don't know if that means changes for individual physicians, or groups, or institutions. The way a physician deals with third party payers has already changed significantly in the last five years. It's very hard to see a patient and make a diagnosis - go through a differential, come to a conclusion over the lab tests, and then just get the data - because right now you call up the third-party carrier and talk to someone who has little or no information. They're the ones who approve the tests or not. I think that kind of third-party intermediary will have to change for medicine to be practiced most effectively. I've seen more occasions where that has interfered with efficient, effective practice of medicine than helped.*

A urologist, accustomed to thinking medically and strategically, sparked an animated conversation with his colleagues by calling them "vendors":

> *This is an interesting one because I think in many ways it is developing strategic business partnerships. I think 'vendor' is an offensive term. Physicians use that. You are vendors. Physicians, as part of the backlash against managed care, are saying that basically all managed care is bad. But what they're really saying is the managed care that attempts to micro-manage, to deny therapy, to limit patient options, may not be the managed care they want. If you look at the basic themes of managed care, I think many of them are very, very admirable.*
>
> *The concept of population management, ambulatory care, studying outcomes, standardizing care, preventive care, providing service, all are terrific, terrific measures. I think people confuse managed care with financing managed care. Whether it's a modified fee for service with withholds or a capitated environment should be secondary. The primary issue should be to determine if this is a rational approach from an individual patient as well as a population measure to a care process moving us away from episodes of illness towards proactive primary care.*

Survey Question 12
How will the digital economy impact the healthcare delivery system?

Unraveling and Re-Birth

Eight physicians representing clinics and hospitals sat together in a focus group wrapping their minds around the digital future and shared their conclusions and apprehensions:

A: The digital economy will encourage the borderline alternative medicine. It may force us to become more accessible to that demand that will be out there through telecommunication. Things like Ask a Nurse *or* Dial a Nurse *may in effect cause loss of money to doctors and hospitals. They can give excellent advice, but that can keep patients from coming into the doctor or the ER.. As long as we are paid per encounter, these services can have a negative financial impact. However, if we go to a capitated payment, the digital economy will be a boon. The digital economy impact depends on what happens to the overall payment scheme.*

B: It just adds more pressure. It's another way of looking at refinement of details and raising expectations. It raises the expectations of patients and payers. How do you provide greater and greater detail, and yet cut down on service and reimbursement? How much more do you expect the doctors to do for less and less? It's just a matter of society saying that 'we have greater degrees of refinement and expectations and we're going to measure you by these greater degrees and expectations, and if you have even a smaller degree of variability you're no longer acceptable.' It just adds external pressures and expectations and it makes the profession less desirable for a physician working in that environment. You don't necessarily get better quality of medicine by refining those measurements. The quality of the measurement and what you're measuring may or may not be accurate. Treating more people, not less. We must make fewer mistakes.

C: A vision for healthcare? Tailor the system to the individual, and not the individual to the system. Patients and their problems are unique. If we don't treat them as individuals and tailor their care, ultimately we won't be giving them the best care, and they won't be satisfied and will go elsewhere.

D: One example might be instead of home visits by a nurse, a computer will be able to do a status check on their condition. This is happening in some places. It's a cost-saving measure, but it removes the personal touch, and there is no way to measure the impact of that on patient care and quality of care.

Survey and Responses

> E: *Healthcare is going in the opposite direction from specialized and customized to one-size-fits-all health care. Healthcare provision is standardized, and when you're an exception to the standard, it's hard to get through the system.*
>
> F: *One caution with healthcare becoming more specialized is that the consumer may expect it to be very individualized, but there is a gap between resources and expectations.*
>
> *So the whole concept of accessing information through the Internet, would that be considered digital economy? Right now we have one of the largest rollouts of a composite medical record. It's a project called Spectrum that we're doing with IBM and Southwestern Bell, Motorola, and Kodak. What this project provides is that doctors at home have access basically to all patient information, including digitized radiological studies, laboratory pharmacy consultant notes. I think that increasingly that type of information, whether it's acquired in the ambulatory environment or hospital environment, will be critical for the ongoing care of patients. But I think, also, medical information will come to doctors differently.*
>
> *I think clinical paths, for example, may become part of a digitized system that, if you prescribe a group of drugs and they're either not as effective as they should be, or they're higher cost, or they otherwise are not appropriate, you would get a real-time, on-line alert to that. So, I think that we'll see a lot more databases, a lot of pieces of information becoming part of a centralized database and a lot of information flowing from that including care paths. Hal Molley actually had an idea for films that he worked on with Sony about eight years ago, interactive videos for patients to make some very tough decisions about breast-sparing surgery, about coronary arteries surgery versus medical management. I mean real tough issues. But they found very quickly that it was not effective unless a skilled professional was leading the patient. That shows that in spite of digital capability and tremendous information available, unsophisticated care recipients will still need to see physicians and other healthcare professionals to access their care.*

Survey Question 13

What other issues do you see impacting healthcare in the future?

Free range. Our respondents offered bullet point answers to this question:
- Provide health care for all.
- Tough economy issues: moral, ethical, and legal.
- Keep personal calling to medicine alive.
- How to care for people where you are, and not be financially incentivized.
- Doing some procedures will cost me (any Doc) more money, a dilemma.
- Invent a new system that is outcome based.
- More women are entering the medical field. Many will be having children.
- We haven't thought about the impact on manpower with maternity leave.
- Alternative medicine will be huge in the future.
- The aging of the population will make demands on the system if they remain unhealthy.
- The abandonment of the children in our society, if they're uninsured.
- The gulf will become greater between children of well-off families and those from poor homes.
- Drop-in medicine has the potential to hurt depending on quality control.
- Doctors should be compelled to continue their education and be re-certified.
- Someone will have to take control of physicians competent.
- Doctors will continue to fight with systems and facilities.
- Payers will continue to try to get every single dollar they can out of the system.
- The government will have to be a part of the medical field.
- The government ought to go in full blast.
- It would take a long time to implement socialized medicine.
- We need to have "Family Centered Care."
- We have to understand the variables in the different cultures.
- Leaders might be better appointed rather than elected. It can be a popularity contest with elections.
- New viruses will be appearing.
- Currently, business is attempting to control medicine. From this we will see an emergence of a single quasi-government type organization that will take the place of individual insurance groups and HMOs.

I think the challenge for the future is, first, how to sustain the excellence that we have in the healthcare system here today and, second, how to advance research that will ultimately improve healthcare by preventing diseases. The reason I say this is that all of the efforts to curtail costs have had a detrimental effect upon attracting high quality people into academic careers and our ability to sustain

Survey and Responses

research in many areas. I think that, although we haven't seen a direct impact yet, if the trend continues for the next 10 years, it does not bode well for this nation.

The production of new medications will accelerate. It is possible to screen compounds much more rapidly and there will be enormous numbers of drugs available. Major improvements in diagnostic equipment will be made. However, the price of producing some of these devices will be so high that most patients may not be able to afford their use.

And finally, one respondent pointed out:

A real interesting piece to me is the whole concept of whether healthcare will, in fact, become integrated. Basically, Regina Herzlinger is challenging the premise of health care integration and believing that it's really going to be niches— home care, long-term care facility, or acute care hospital. To me the real question is: Is integration the future of healthcare or is it about basically having the finances of healthcare, the Wall Street model, carve out healthcare so the primary care doctor and many doctors become medical concierges rather than gatekeepers? I don't think gatekeeper is the right approach either. I think it's in what we're building here, how you balance the appropriateness of primary care with the requirements for excellence in sub-specialty care.

Aside from their sharing of ideas, the physicians reported that it was great fun thinking together about new paradigms and comparing notes with colleagues. One remarked: "This felt like medical school again. I love the challenge of thinking differently about old topics and discovering things for the first time."

Chapter 4our

Learning Disabilities in HealthCare Systems

The ten learning disabilities discovered and uncovered in healthcare systems is present in nearly every system, regardless of size or location. Larger systems with an employee population of 10,000 and above are more likely to experience nearly all of the disabilities. Small systems report much less internal competition, or administrative splits.

1. Fragmentation
2. Polarization
3. Fear of future
4. Suspect relationship with communities
5. Turnover of staff
6. Too much management, not enough leadership
7. Medical Arms Race
8. Destructive internal competition
9. Reactive behaviors at all levels
10. Split between administrators and physicians

1. Fragmentation

Fragmentation is another way of describing disintegration. Several of the systems included in the study have a history of cooperation, collaboration, and careful attention to cross-functionality with an intense focus on the patient. For some, things began to change in the mid-80s with mergers of systems, particularly of hospitals with dissimilar values. Systems became larger, purchased clinics and wrapped them into 'dissimilarity' where the patient became a number and the physician became a 'provider'.

Physicians became disenfranchised, and the system became Satanic to them. Departments became separate business units, looking at other departments as competitors for resources, personnel and market share. The bottom line became the focus even as the language

Learning Disabilities

changed. Administrators spoke businessese, physicians spoke medicalese, department heads held unitized meetings that involved other departments without inviting impacted parties. What began as 'save you rear-end' meetings ended in warfare where bunkers were designed with clear boundaries and weaponry.

Communication was more than a challenge. It became nearly impossible. "Why should we talk with the enemy? Find out what they're doing and make sure we get everything first. Send in the spies. Get close to the people with the money. Look nice if you have to, even smile, but beat them!" For purposes of publication, this is a highly cleaned up version of what actually was said and what happened.

We witnessed departmental meetings, faculty sessions where department heads and deans (of medical schools) engaged in shouting matches between physicians, physicians and administrators. Attempting to negotiate a different way to think about healthcare delivery, or new ways to create a learning environment for medical students, became intellectual and emotional warfare. Social astuteness, the skill that measures the ability to read verbal and non-verbal behavior, was (and perhaps still is) conspicuous by its deficiency and absence.

Fragmentation is perhaps the most debilitating disability since the outcome is disintegration. The causes for fragmentation are:

Defensiveness
Denial
Defamation
Delay
Depart

Defensiveness arises out of anger and judgment. When seemingly innocent questions begin with WHY, the pursuit is on behalf of inflicting pain and not the acquisition of information.

Denial is the attempt to avoid accountability and/or blame and thus lie in order to preserve falsehoods.

Defamation is vilification often disguised as 'left handed' acclaim. It is slander, backbiting, and libel wrapped in the language of pity.

Delay is the activity of passive-aggressive wannabees or people who dislike any kind of truth telling.

Departing is the aggressive behavior of those who cut and run in the face of stress, potential criticism, and adverse public opinion.

2. Polarization.

Divergence of opinions, goals, values, and beliefs happens when there is no will to listen or converse while suspending judgment.

We discovered polarization between primary care physicians and physician specialists, between physicians and nurses, between physicians and administrators, between administrators and regulators, between educators and students.

The absence of respect for differences, the unwillingness to learn from one another, the cognitive inability to look at root causes, and the emotional inability to examine personal, professional, and organizational behavior all contribute to predictable polarization.

The polarization we discovered was caused by the basic human factors of wanting credit rather than sharing it; wanting center stage rather than sharing it; wanting to be heard rather than listening; wanting to exclude, not include; wanting to hear confessions of omission and commission and not confessing and holding confession as weapons of intimidation and manipulation; wanting to be served instead of serving. This is the breeding ground of persuasive, pitiful, polarization.

3. Fear

Fear of the future is another way of talking about worry. Worry is and can be crippling, stress inducing, resulting in personal and organizational disability. Listen to the voices.

Our research uncovered a variety of fears impacting every level of healthcare including:

Fear of the future. "Who will buy us next week?" "Will I have a job?" "I've had three supervisors in six months? Am I the next to go?" In 1996 there were 167 hospital mergers. That number increased by 21.6% in 1997 with 203 mergers according to the Hospital Acquisition Report, Fourth Edition. But while the number of mergers increased, the number of hospital involved in those transactions actually declined. That figure dropped from 323 hospitals involved in mergers in 1996 to 276 in 1997, a 14.6% decrease.

Learning Disabilities

Stephen Monroe, a partner at Irving Levin, noted that while the merger trend continues, "there has been an increase in the single hospital merger or acquisition as opposed to the large chain mergers of a few years ago. More community hospitals are deciding that it is too risky to remain independent in today's world of managed care and are seeking partners."

The report also demonstrated a shift in the type of purchasers in the hospital market. In 1997, non-profit hospital companies were the purchasers in 75% of the transactions, and those acquisitions represented 73% of the hospitals bought during the year. "A few years ago, the for-profit hospital chains were expanding rapidly through acquisition," Monroe said. "Now, it is the non-profits who have dominated the market for the past two years."

Fear of failure. "There's no room for mistakes around here. We make mistakes and can't admit to it. We are told to shut up so we don't get sued."

Fear of not making budget. "We used to put the patient first; now we put the budget first. The boss around here is money. We hear 'no margin, no mission'. It's like a mantra. We don't hear anyone saying, 'no patients, no work.'"

Fear of saying the wrong thing. "One of our values is so-called fearless communication. That's a joke! Speak your mind around here and you're on the street. Isn't falsehood the real jail? Why are people so afraid of the truth? I'm afraid because I need my job; my kids need to eat and nobody is willing to pay the mortgage."

4. Relationship with the community

Historically, hospitals and clinics were nearly beyond reproach. Now we can access the Internet, Associated Press, Trade Journals, and the hometown weekly paper and read of fraud, lawsuits because of incompetence, license revocation, and penalties because of inadequate care.

The public is questioning both private, church held and public healthcare institutions as never before. Development officers in healthcare are finding it a major challenge to raise money for bricks and mortar. One bad clinic, one deposed physician, one nursing home indicted for neglect, taints everyone. The public has become less forgiving of incompetence, neglect, and suspect accountability.

Unraveling and Re-Birth

The fragmentation, polarization, and fear that one resided inside healthcare organizations, has become public. The public trust has been violated. Credibility of healthcare institutions is no long automatic.

5. Turnover of staff

The following add on the Internet regarding long term care is sobering and documented.

Do You Have Reasons To Be Concerned About Long Term Care? Until you can feel comfortable about applying for long term care insurance, you must understand the risk of needing long-term care. If you're one who thinks you'll ever need long term care, take a peak at the following statistics: There's a 43% chance that a person 65 years or older will eventually enter a nursing home sometime during their lifetime. [1]

A year in a nursing home now averages more than $52,000, and can exceed $100,000 in some parts of the country.[2]

Most nursing home stays are about two-and-a-half years.[3]

It's estimated that 7 in 10 people will use home care. [4]

Approximately 22.4 million families are involved in long-term in-home care. [5]

About 41 of every 1,000 Americans over 65 are in nursing homes. [6]

[1] Working Woman, 9/97, [2]. The Wall Street Journal, 3/31/99 [3].The Boston Globe, 5/12/97, [4]. Business Week, 7/20/98, [5]. USA Today, 3/18/97, [6]. Business Week 2/17/97.

It's easy to pick on the industry that has more regulations governing it than the atomic energy commission. Long-term care work is difficult at best. Commonly heard in nursing homes from certified nursing assistants is "Why should I work with difficult residents/patients when I can flip hamburgers for $.50 an hour more?"

What is there a nursing shortage? Why do some healthcare systems experience more than 50% turnover in staff annually? The staff survey for this study indicated that turnover begins with the warning signs of burnout, which is substantiated in Nurseweek Magazine 2/97.

Learning Disabilities

Physical Signs	Emotional Signs	Behavioral
Clammy hands	Anxiety	Blaming others
Diarrhea	Discouragement and depression	Crying
Dry mouth	Fear	Irritability
Eating disorders	Frustration	Short attention span
Heart palpitations	Powerlessness	Short temper
Halitosis	Grief	Over activity
Stiffness	Feeling worthless	Risk taking
Back pain	Isolation	Negative attitude

The Healthcare Association of southern California examined the turnover and shortage problems in California with the following results:

About 50% of RNs registered are educated outside of the state.

Most racial/ethnic groups are underrepresented among RNs. The gap is most pronounced for Hispanics, who account for 30% of the population, but only 4% of the state's RNs.

Nurses are aging along with the rest of the population. Less than 10% are younger than 30 ears old. The average age is in the upper 40s. About one-third are older than age 50, and 15% are more than 60 years old.

By 2010, more than 40% of the nursing work force will be older than age 50. California's population is surging and projected to grow from 32.5 million to 49.23 million between 2000 and 2025.

Enrollments in bachelor's-degree nursing programs have declined consistently over the past five years nationwide, dropping 4.6% in 1999 alone, according to the latest annual survey by the American Association of Colleges of Nursing.

The Bureau of Labor Statistics projects a 12.5% increase in RN hospital positions by 2005. However, as a percentage of total RN jobs in all settings, RN hospital jobs will decrease from 64% to 57%.

Burnout, shortage, aging work population, and fear because of potential job loss, all contribute to turnover.

6. Too much management, not enough leadership

Healthcare systems are complex. "Management is about coping with complexity", writes John Kotter (Harvard Business Review 6/90). "Leadership, by contrast, is about coping with change."

Complexity is managed by budgeting, planning, organizing, staffing, and controlling. Leadership involves vision, values, inspiration, credibility, communication, and setting the right direction. Management is concerned about managing stuff while leadership is concerned about insuring significance. Many of the healthcare systems involved in this study may be over managed and under led.

7. Medical Arms Race

In many of the major cities where this study was conducted, there is visible evidence of how money is thrown at equipment in order to 'stay competitive'.

Through e-health, a patient in the U.S. or anywhere in the world could undergo magnetic resonance imaging, an X-ray or other diagnostic test in his or her own country and have it read via the Internet at a Canadian doctor's computer screen, for a fee. Other services could involve Canadian doctors' consulting physicians in other countries via the Internet.

There are, for example, more magnetic resonance imaging (MRI) machines in the Twin Cities of Minneapolis and St. Paul, that in the entire country of Canada. The same is true for the city of Baltimore and other major cities.

Hospital and clinic presidents/administrators interviewed wondered where and when the race will stop. Is collective collaboration in the utilization of expensive medical equipment irrelevant? Hospital A purchases expensive equipment because Hospital B is having identical equipment installed. And the costs spiral.

8. Destructive Internal Competition

Competition is here to stay, regardless of the political dimensions of the nation or the organization. Competition by definition is one opponent against another, antagonism, struggle, a contest. Competition is expected between and among companies and organizations that have the same or similar products and services. The problem is when the antagonism and struggle becomes an internal contest for resources, recognition, respect, and individual or departmental rewards.

Learning Disabilities

Many of our respondents linked destructive internal competition with the 'bunker' mentality that exists between sections, units, and departments in hospitals, larger systems, and even small clinics.

The destructive competition often begins and ends with the budgeting process. Political maneuvering, persuasive debate, veiled threats, and outright lies become the force, not power that is exerted to exact selfish gain. That's destructive internal competition.

9. Reactive Behaviors At All Levels

Healthcare in general and medical practice specifically, is seldom proactive. There has been considerable conversation in the last decade about prevention and wellness. There was little debate among those surveyed and interviewed about the fact that medical education in many of our medical schools operates on an academic formula, which supports the illness model, not wellness.

The question is: who takes the initiative in healthcare?

The patient? The physician? The system? Regulators? Insurers? There is considerable press about healthcare being broken. Who is responsible for the brokenness? Finger pointing and assigning blame is not likely to fix a broken system. Our interviewed respondents suggest that we are spending considerable time, money, and energy fixing a broken chariot. There are, as many report, no horses strong enough to pull it through the mud of competition, indecision, political intrigue, or mindless optimism.

10. Split between physicians and administrators

The chasm between physicians and administrators is evident on several fronts: language, attitude, and orientation.

Language. Administrators use language common to MBA graduates: delegation, budget, cost analysis and containment, control, debt ratios, FTEs, etc. Physicians use language, especially medical shorthand known only by physicians and certain allied staff which is often perceived by administrators as in-house code for keeping administrators at bay.

Attitude. Many administrators struggle with how to deal with feeling second class to physicians who may feel superior because of education, place in the food chain, prestige among professionals, among other social stratification criteria. The competitive relationship is often unproductive, unnecessary, and unwanted. Many hope for a gain/gain relationships where respect is alive and well together with appropriate division of labor where credit is shared and celebrated.

Orientation. The orientation of many administrators is clearly on numbers – revenue, staffing, profit, debt, reserves, and investments. Physicians are oriented to patient care, to diagnosis and treatment, to healing and being fairly compensated. Administrators we've heard, say, "I don't understand them. Why don't they attempt to learn about what I do and why. They're only concerned about their corner of the world." Physicians we've heard, say "Administrators! Who needs 'em? They wouldn't have a job without us."

Fortunately, the chasm between them can be crossed. Healthy healthcare systems have found ways to build bridges between these two worlds. The sad thing about this disability is that it is taken for granted by both parties.

Learning disabilities are present in every organization. Healthcare systems have the additional burden and challenge of addressing them since everyone appears to be an expert regarding healthcare delivery. The public is vested in healthcare and expects the best delivery system in the world to be much better than it is. We know what is good and want it to be better. Patients are not interested in the internal squabbles between physicians or the seemingly adolescent behavior between competing systems. Patients want caring, competent, complete, careful, cost-effective, clinically up-to-date healthcare. Patients are becoming more demanding and informed. God does not wear a white jacket adorned by long necklace, often used as a tool.

So, who's coming to the table? Hundreds of respondents asked, "How long will it take for healthcare stakeholders to park their pride and arrogance at the door and enter the negotiation room with humility and strong wills?" Weeds are growing on the road less traveled.

Learning Disabilities

"Good judgment comes from experience,
and experience
comes from bad judgment."

-Barry LePatner

Chapter 5ive

Competencies of the Physician Leader

Perceptions of physician executives are reflected in the informal labels given to them by others. First, their straightforward, formal titles:

- Executive Vice President of Medical Affairs
- Vice President of Medical Affairs
- Chief Medical Officer
- Director of Medical Affairs
- Medical Director
- Chief of Medical Affairs

In contrast, their informal names imply various and derogatory things. There are physicians who dislike anything that smacks of management. They use these labels to show their disdain for someone with the power to direct their medical practice or influence their future.

- Big Medical Kahuna
- The Suit
- The P & P Doc
- The Management Guy/Gal
- Him
- Her

These titles for physician executives help identify the obstacles and demanding expectations they face in their roles.

Big Medical Kahuna. A Big Medical Kahuna is expected to be a walking, talking, stalking encyclopedia of medical protocols, policies, and procedures, with the ability to articulate it all on command while monitoring the work of both the worst and the best of attending physicians.

The Suit. The Suit is the non-complimentary name given to the physician who has deserted the ranks of practicing physicians in favor of the executive suite. Those who avoid the title of "The Suit" are physician executives who continue to practice while wearing the suit. Many physicians have a knee-jerk distaste for management or those who want to manage.

Competencies

The P & P Doc. The P & P Doc, who is mainly concerned with policies and procedures, tends to want to exercise control. Since most physicians practice self-control, and since most management policies have more to do with management than with the practice of medicine, the P & P Doc frequently is resisted or ignored.

The Management Guy/Gal/Him/Her. This term is similar to The Suit. Many physicians conclude that other physicians elevated to the rank of chief medical officer are those who can't make it anywhere else. While this conclusion is usually unwarranted and unfair, it is nonetheless a perception that physician executives must deal with. Most physicians who are chief medical officers have demonstrated the ability to practice outstanding medicine and, usually through their communication and negotiation skills in difficult situations, to represent their peers. Often derogatory attitudes toward them come from those who'd like to represent other physicians even though they haven't demonstrated the "currency" to be chosen for the position.

One of my intents in this book is to help frame the new role and responsibility of physician executives and leaders by debugging bias, challenging new ways to think about leadership, and declaring war on attitudes of entitlement and victimization.

Competencies of a Successful Physician Leader

To be successful, physician leaders need to be qualified, competent, ready, and fit—across a number of dimensions. Personnel Decisions International (PDI) has researched and developed a comprehensive leadership competencies model for physician leaders. These address expected standards of performance for the contemporary and future physician. To be truly effective in the changing organizational environments of the healthcare industry, that physician must actively pursue, and participate in, the creative decision-making needed to reinvent healthcare.

Competency models form the foundation for integrated performance management and development strategies (which may include, for instance, assessment centers, 360-degree feedback instruments and processes, targeted training, and individual coaching) related to specific professions and industries. In 1991, the Healthcare Forum undertook a study of leadership practices in healthcare organizations. Respondents were asked to rate 36 leadership competencies with respect to their current prevalence and future importance. Their ratings and additional data from a number of similar studies, together with validation studies of its specific models, support PDI's identification of given competencies.

PDI's generic competencies model for physician leaders is customized for individual healthcare clients. This chapter presents samples of competencies and related behaviors drawn from the generic and customized models. (Any PDI office has information on English models and the availability of translated versions.)

Foundational Leadership Skills and Attributes (Note: Each competency is supported by up to ten descriptive items, which give specificity to it. We offer one item as a sample here.)

Visionary Thinking	Sees future possibilities and anticipates their implications.
System-Oriented Thinking	Looks at problems and issues from a holistic perspective
Speaking with Impact	Communicates views and presents ideas in a clear and convincing manner.
Fostering Open Dialogue	Facilitates open, two-way communication among individuals and groups.
Listening	Demonstrates attention to and conveys understanding of the comments and questions of others.
Inspiring Trust	Conducts oneself with integrity, professional ethics, and fairness, and demonstrates the courage of strong convictions.
Building Relationships	Builds an active network of mutually beneficial relationships both within and outside the organization.

Competencies

Managing Disagreements	Brings conflicts and disagreements into the open and works to resolve them collaboratively.
Developing Others	Shares personal expertise to help others grow and develop.
Professional Credibility	Commands the respect of colleagues based on professional achievements.
Customer/Patient Focus	Anticipates customer/patient needs; takes action to meet customer/patient needs; continually searches for ways to increase customer/patient satisfaction.
Adaptability/ Resourcefulness	Maintains a constructive attitude and approach in response to change, pressure, and adversity.
Working Efficiently	Organizes own and others' work for greatest efficiency.
Promoting Diversity	Shows and fosters respect and appreciation for all individuals regardless of values, perspectives, and interests in order to enhance business decisions.
Inspiring Commitment	Presents ideas and recommendations persuasively and gains support and commitment to collective action.
Strategic Talent Development	Identifies, attracts, and develops the best talent in the field.
Developing Teams/Teamwork	Builds effective teams and fosters teamwork across the organization.
Business Acumen	Recognizes the full range of business principles that impact the healthcare industry, and obtains/applies the appropriate resources to achieve integration of clinical and business goals.
Service Excellence	Continually strives to meet the needs and exceed the expectations of patients and other internal and external customers.
Clinical Process Improvement	Promotes clinical care (e.g., diagnosis, treatment) as a set of processes with opportunities for systematic improvement.
Clinical Vision/Innovation	Demonstrates a clear vision for clinical care and a desire to develop innovative approaches to clinical care.
Clinical/Patient Advocacy	Champions the view that patient health and welfare are the reasons for all health care

	processes.
Strategic Vision	Establishes compelling goals and develops effective strategies and plans to achieve them.
Seasoned Judgment	Makes well-reasoned, timely decisions based on practical experience and sound logic.
Organization Alignment	Organizes resources and builds alliances to achieve strategic goals and increase efficiency.
Managing for Results	Assigns accountability, coordinates efforts, and follows through to ensure that results are achieved.

The Transition

The transition from clinical practice to physician executive leadership, particularly for the Medical Director or the VP of Medical Affairs, can be difficult and disorienting. The transition involves changes:

—from independent to a dependent orientation
—in focus from patient to organization
—of role from control to influence and persuasion
—in relationships to colleague from peer to overseer
—from a medical to a business mindset

These changes are compounded by the fact that most physicians distrust management. Impressed more by medical achievements than administrative acumen, physicians have little respect for anyone who has moved from an orientation of quality to an orientation of cost containment and what they experience as "administrivia."[37] The challenges for the physician leader and physician executive can be intense emotionally. Most new physician executives are ill prepared to deal with the distrust of other physicians.

Many physicians, like many people in general, dislike certain behaviors in others that they see in themselves. Chief among these are arrogance and insensitivity. The physician contributors to this volume noted that most physicians have little interest or skill in choosing or

Competencies

managing a staff, adapting to anyone in a position of authority, dealing productively with conflict, or the ability to delegate.

A naive conclusion made by physicians about physician executives is that the executives have "sold out." Or, they might think, "I can't do it; I don't understand it and, therefore, don't see any value in it." A physician contemplating a move into a position of formal leadership or management must be aware of subtle and concealed potholes, as well as overt and sometimes hostile attitudes. Potholes include a silent treatment, a smiling distance, a passive-aggressive acceptance, and an attitude expressing something like, "We got along just fine before you arrived. Why don't you go back to being a real doctor?"

The Dilemma of the Physician Leader/Executive

The Magician. The *Now-You-See-It-Now-You-Don't* magicians' club threw a holiday party. A magician from another club was invited to be the stand-up entertainer. The entertainment was a bust. The illusions didn't impress the audience. They knew all the tricks. There were snide remarks, "Did you see that? My kids can do better. Did he think he could really put that one over on us?"

When physicians become physician executives and they try to motivate others with motivational techniques, those other physicians recognize the techniques being used on them. Like the magicians at the party, they see through the illusions of leadership if and when it is disingenuous; its effect is lost on them. They see right off that the emperor has no clothes.

Physicians dislike managing and being managed. However, to lead is not the same as to manage. Physician executives must decide if they want to be, primarily, a leader or a manager, and when to lead and when to manage. Their more fundamental, related decision is determining how they really want to participate in the medical community, that is, what they want to bring to that community—not what they want to get from it.

If a physician executive wants primarily to bring greater efficiency and cost containment to their enterprise, then s/he is choosing the role of the manager. If s/he chooses to develop the people and the organization in order to serve patients better, then s/he is choosing the role of leader. Until a richer, more integrated leadership role for the physician executive is fully accepted, the managerial role will tend to pit efficiency and cost containment against patient care. Physician executives fulfilling a richer, more integrated leadership role would:

- be accessible and friendly
- put the interests of others before their own
- deal concretely and creatively with problems and issues
- take the short and long-term view
- be self-confident and confront and support all internal champions
- value and maintain high trust levels
- know which battles to fight and which to ignore
- be at home with clinical and administrative language and concepts
- be adept, using models and paradigms appropriate to the situation, person, or group
- know what is really going on, personally, professionally and organizationally

Physician executives become *ineffective* when they:

- are aloof or arrogant
- follow self-centered ambition
- fail to deal with issues and problems
- take only the short-term view
- are dependent on an internal political champion
- betray trust
- are overly involved or interested in administrative detail
- drop clinical language in favor of administrative language
- do not recognize different situations, thinking that one size fits all
- show little or no flexibility and adeptness
- deny, avoid and escape tough realities
- fail to link personal, professional and organization savvy

Adeptness and Learning

Effective leaders have learned to cooperate, collaborate, and adapt. Those who compete as individuals are warriors fighting the wrong battles. The only warriors needed in healthcare are those battling disease or championing the cause of their patients. As for their adeptness into the future, physician executives need to build a range of new technical and non-technical skills. Specific skill areas addressed here are information technology, communication, relationships,

Competencies

negotiation, teamwork, organizational politics, dealing with the patient's family, physicians' generation gap, dealing with different work style types, physician interaction styles, and conflict management.

Information technology. An endocrinologist skilled in his specialty and conversant on information technology systems is aware of the need to unite medicine with technology:

Computer literacy, MIS systems, and high tech charting. We must learn to access information that is available on the Internet. Physicians have to stay current on all of the technical advances as they rise in their specialties. They need to know what is useful and what is a waste of time. There are ways to get data quickly and that is good; this is where we will be able to access much of the research in the future.

Communication. A plastic surgeon with an appetite for reading is critical of his colleagues who seldom read or write:

Most of my colleagues don't read anything other than an occasional journal article from our trade magazines like JAMA or the New England Journal. I could go to the offices of 20 of my physician friends and find a computer on the desks of five or six. A visit to their homes reveals nice looking libraries filled with unread books. When asked about the dust on the books, I hear excuses about time. Communication skills are very important. I developed my skills reading the masters and patterning my writing skills after the best. Physicians need to be on the cutting edge of their field and know what is the best and most cost-effective approach to a particular problem. With the focus on cost and quality, physicians will be under a magnifying glass. Learning to keep up with one's discipline will be an increasing challenge, and we can't keep up with dust on our books or by being afraid of a box on the desk.

Relationships. A forensic pathologist knew that he didn't understand much about human relationships, so he found a mentor to help him with his interpersonal skills. He spoke with confidence.

In the non-technical area, it involves the people skills—enhancing intense relationships with patients, managerial skills, the ability to do consensus building and collaboration and to understand that you're going to have to work with other things. If we're going to be successful, we're going to have to develop ways of reaching out to the community and to hear the community voices. Not saying 'We think you need this, and that's what you're going to get.' There have to be mechanisms, not only in the workplace, but also in networking, and by mechanisms—I mean CME courses that have impact.

Negotiation. A public health physician said:

Negotiation requires a different set of skills than what physicians typically are trained in and a different sensitivity, too. There needs to be more explanation. We can't say, 'I know what's best for you, please don't question it, just take this pill it's going to make you feel better.' We need to give patients a choice. They need to be informed so they can make decisions about their futures. Physicians will need to be able to involve patients in the decision-making process. Patients are more knowledgeable, they ask more questions, and they will have opinions about their treatment. This creates a challenge and a need for physicians to have negotiation skills.

Teams. A doctor spoke sensitively to the need for more team behavior:

Physicians will have to be better team members. Relationships with nurses, other physicians, hospitals, etc., will be more important. Executives need to have knowledge of finance, operations management, marketing, and organizational behavior. In any situation it's important to understand what the underlying problem is, and what impact a range of different possible solutions likely will have. Ever wonder why so many physicians have trouble with head nurses or directors of nursing? Nurses know how to play occupational team sports while most physicians play occupational ping-pong.

Politics. Politics is a combat sport in healthcare while people who are political tend to be mistrusted. Physicians who occupy the office of medical director or the vice president of medical affairs or even the CEO of a hospital or healthcare system are politically suspect. Non-executive physicians say, "Can I trust him/her now? Will I hear what they think I want to hear? Is s/he singing a tune given by the board or is it the truth? I'll wait around and do my own testing."

In the past, medical directors were elected by consensus - that's changing. Recently, flawed selection processes occurred, such as: "Let's elect Harry since he's close to retirement." Or, "Get Pat who will do the least harm." The American Medical Directors Association

Competencies

(AMDA) has established principles for electing or selecting a medical director. AMDA is responsible for a rigorous certification program developed together with substantive continuing medical education requirements. There are new rules, especially in the long-term care industry.

Consensus can be a problem in the healthcare industry. It has contributed to organizational black holes and groupthink. It can protect any system from change, keep incompetent managers in their offices, insure stability for the fearful, protect a hierarchy's static order, and result in mindless homogeneity. It does not encourage us to look at the whole picture. On the other hand, consensus can allow us to work in non-destructive boredom, offer life without revolution in the midst of ongoing change, permit us to watch progress from a stalled train, and build and support socialized medicine or free-market medicine

Physician leaders must be acutely aware of the landmines of politicized medicine. The hundreds of physicians I interviewed typically were open, candid, and irreverently forthright. Politicized medicine will dampen that spirit, will affect the quality of medical education and care in our hospitals, clinics, and nursing homes. Physician leaders have the burden of maintaining interpersonal openness and guarding organizational integrity.

Family. Experienced in dealing with emergencies and difficult situations, an emergency physician spoke with authority:

Dealing with families and family systems is important, but often not taken into account. Doctors need to realize that they are not dealing with one individual patient, but a member of a family system that may or may not be affecting the patient's physical health. In the case of terminally ill patients, dealing with the whole family is critical, but we are not trained in medical school to deal with this issue. Medical schools and instructors are challenged to teach the competencies necessary to deal with families, not just patients. The bedside covers every square foot of the hospital.

Physicians' generation gap. A 61-year-old family physician said:

There are generational and motivational gaps between physicians. The old-school physician was expected to be on call every third night, and to stay at the hospital until wee hours in the morning, until a patient improved. Now, the younger docs are more concerned with getting out of the hospital as soon as possible. They are concerned with the quality of their life and their hobbies. They look at this as a job, rather than a calling. There is an

Unraveling and Re-Birth

increasing war between the two groups and to manage it within a clinic is a major challenge.

Dealing with different work style types. Physician executives need to understand themselves, their own work styles, and the work styles of others. The Myers-Briggs Type Indicator (MBTI), for example, can help. It is a neutral inventory that describes 16 different work style types and associated preferences based on four continuums: (1) introversion and extroversion; (2) sensing and intuition; (3) thinking and feeling; (4) judging and perceiving. Individuals' responses to the inventory questions reveal their individual type.

While some work style types and associated preferences clearly support a leadership role, others do not. A physician understands this about himself:

> *I am a technocrat trained in anatomic pathology. There will be a definite role for physician technocrats in the healthcare environment, but not in a leadership role. A technocrat has characteristics unsuitable for leadership positions such as perfectionism; defensiveness under explicit or implicit criticism; preoccupation with details, rules, lists, orders, systems, schedules. Technocrats are usually organized around dominance and submission and insist on their own way, and they assume that superior intelligence equates with good judgment. They avoid impulsiveness, are emotionally distant, and are best suited for responsibilities that don't involve people contact.*

Physician interaction styles. Four styles of physician interaction represent different levels of skill and responsibility in technical and non-technical areas. These are: Technician, Professional, Rookie, and Counselor. A physician who has reached the status of counselor and professional can recognize and manage four conflict strategies—*avoidance, diffusion, containment, confrontation*—with ease and effectiveness. This configuration below accompanies Arnold and Feldman's (*Managing Individual and Group Behavior in Organizations:* McGraw Hill) model of eight conflict management strategies (next page). Together, these can be applied to physician interaction and conflict management within teams and organizations.

Competencies

Technical High	**Technician** Advanced technical skills	**Professional** Advanced interpersonal skills Advanced technical skills	Technician Advanced technical skills
Non- technical Low	**Rookie** Elementary technical & interpersonal skills	**Counselor** Advanced interpersonal skills	Non-technical High

All physicians begin as rookies. Formal and informal medical education contributes to the development of technical skills until the rookie becomes a technician. Next, the residency program enhances technical skills and develops the human, interactive, and interpersonal dimensions of physicians for their role of counselor. After considerable experience they reach the professional level in which they serve as expert, counselor, leader, coach, respected colleague, and sought after physician. A competent physician is a life-long learner who is ready to acknowledge and deal with chaos and uncertainty.

Conflict Management. Physicians care deeply about many things. When Dr. Jones cares deeply about a procedure that has worked successfully and Dr. Brown introduces a new procedure that denigrates in effect Dr. Jones's work, conflict arises. Interpersonal and intergroup conflict can arise out of caring, confrontation, or callous disregard. The following typology may assist in guiding serious conversations and behaviors to deal constructively with conflict.

Conflict Resolution Strategy	Type of Strategy	Appropriate Situations
Ignoring the conflict	Avoidance	When the issue is trivial; when the issue is symptomatic of mere basic, pressing problems
Imposing a solution	Avoidance	When quick, decisive action is needed; when unpopular decisions need to be made and consensus among the groups appears very unlikely
Smoothing	Diffusion	As a stopgap measure to let people cool down and regain perspective; when the conflict is over non-work issues
Appealing to super-ordinate goals	Diffusion	When there is a mutually important goal that neither group can achieve without the cooperation of the other, when the survival or success of the overall organization is in jeopardy

Bargaining	Containment	When the two parties are of relatively equal power; when there are several acceptable, alternative solutions that both parties would be willing to consider
Structuring the interaction	Containment	When previous attempts to openly discuss conflict issues led to conflict escalation rather than to problem solution; when a respected third party is available to provide some structure and could serve as a mediator
Integrative problem solving	Confrontation	When there is a minimum level of trust between groups and there is no time pressure for a quick solution; when the organization can benefit from merging the differing perspectives and insights of the groups in making key decisions
Redesigning the organization	Confrontation	When the sources of conflict come from the coordination of work; when the work can be easily divided into clear project responsibilities (self-contained work groups); when activities require a lot of interdepartmental coordination over time (lateral relations)

An Overview of Points on Physicians and Physician Executives

Common tendencies for the physician leader to overcome:

- Physicians are trained to respond with, not anticipate, interventions (they are more reactive than proactive).
- Physicians dislike being managed.
- Physicians entering management are inadequately prepared to adopt and implement effective management practices and techniques.
- The skills required in effective management often contradict and sometimes negate the skills learned in patient care.
- Physicians move into management for one or more of their following desires to:

—pursue personal growth and challenge

—develop new policies and change the system

—improve the quality of patient care

—influence and lead others as an administrator

Competencies

—have an impact on a larger audience

—reduce job stress

—receive greater financial remuneration

—relieve boredom with clinical practice

—allow for more personal time

General differences between clinicians and managers. The common tendencies for physician leaders to overcome have parallels in how clinicians' professional role differs from that of managers, as follows:

Clinicians ↓	*Managers/Leaders* ↓
Doers	Planners, designers
Reactive personalities	**Proactive personalities**
Require immediate gratification	Accept delayed gratification
Deciders: often decides alone	**Delegators: uses teamwork**
Value autonomy	Value collaboration
Independent	Participative
Patient advocate	Organization advocate
Identify with profession	**Identify with organization**
Think in clinical terms	Think in organization/business terms
Risk aversive	**Risk takers**
One-to-one interaction(s)	One-on-one interaction(s)
Control	**Control**
Short term horizon	Long term vision
Perfectionism	**Gradual improvement**
Empathic	Objective & Intuitive
Quality oriented	**Cost-oriented**
Certainty	Uncertainty, ambiguity
Patient dependency	**Partnership**
Fragmentation (specialty)	Systems view
Self-definition	**Part of a larger whole**
Saving lives	Healing self and community
Personal responsibility	**Shared responsibility**
Autonomy	Collaboration
Deductive reasoning	**Deductive & inductive reasoning**
Identity as MD	Identity linked to organization

Behavioral profiles of physician executives (Source: R.W. Singleton)
- Strong communication skills
- People oriented
- Strong leaders
- Self-motivated
- Industrious

Competencies

- Driven by accomplishments

CEO expectations for physician executive behavior (Source: Seibert & Singleton)

- Seek new ideas and methods of getting results
- Seek and evaluate information before making decisions
- Identify problems, subjects, or priorities needing to be discussed
- Work cooperatively with others to accomplish tasks
- Facilitate interaction between people to achieve results

Professional development needs for physicians

- Management training
- Business education and organizational awareness education
- Team interaction skills
- Collaborative skills

Professional development needs for physician executives

- Manage the information/technology explosion
- Manage physicians who resist change
- Anticipate personnel needs vs. reacting to needs (fire prevention, not fire fighting)
- Sponsor management and interpersonal training needs of care providers and physicians
- Initiate continuing education programs: The Physician as Leader
- Impacting/Influencing the Healthcare System (Organization) as Physician Executive

Chapter 6ix

Power and Leadership

Our understanding of power in organizations is changing dramatically and with good cause. Robert Dilenschneider (Power and Influence: Mastering the Art of Persuasion: Simon & Schuster) has outlined the evolution of organizational power since the 1950s.

Evolution of Power

1950s and 1960s	1970s and 1980s	1990s
Power as Administration	Power as Management	Power as Leadership
Company chain of command	Exception-driven	Visionary
Conformist	Ad hoc	Instant
Stable	Turbulent	Sustaining
Introspective	Market-driven	Positioning
Apprenticeship	Mentoring	Collegial

Dilenschneider's description has to do with the nature, perception, and distribution of decision-making power. Its three eras can be characterized by (1) the military model, (2) the managerial model, and (3) the mutuality model. When power operated as administration in the 50s and 60s, it controlled the organization through orders passed down, reflecting a military model. In the 70s and 80s, decisions were made on the basis of what managers might choose to do in their areas, within top-down constraints. In the 90s, power has been based increasingly on the sharing of goals, decisions, and outcomes among leaders and followers. In terms of decisions, the military model is swift and direct, and it carries clear consequences. The managerial model is arbitrary, focused on need and driven by exception. The mutuality model is more time-consuming, respectful, future oriented, and clearly the model of the future.

Today, a physician leader has options for the ways in which he/she might exercise power in healthcare organizations by:

- Analyzing trends
- Crafting agendas
- Seeking and taking advice

Power and Leadership

- Creating and sustaining a strong vision
- Articulating clear objectives
- Being action oriented
- Training self and others to focus on critical issues
- Harmonizing vision and best practices
- Leveraging the culture of the organization
- Practicing simple and simply profound communication

Individual and Group Trends

Healthcare practitioners, individuals and groups, are facing increased complexity in the healthcare environment. The future demands that physicians, nurses, allied health professionals, administrative executives, and regulators work collaboratively to maximize every identifiable resource. This demand puts a different emphasis on managerial functions. The table charts related trends of the last half of the 20th century.

Individual or Group	Past 1950's-1980s	Present (1990s)	1995 and beyond
Physicians	Solo practice	Group practice	Corporate practice, active involvement in managerial activity
Nurses	Clinical practice	Emerging as a political force	Active participation in managerial structure and policy
Allied Health	Not an issue	Emerging issue	Key participants in teams that manage care across episodes of illness and pathways of wellness
Management research and assessment	Not an issue	Increased recognition	Integral part of managerial, organizational effectiveness
Dynamic nature of groups	Individual & disciplinary groups dominate	Emergence of interdisciplinary groups	Dominance of interdisciplinary groups
Information management	Not an issue	Emerging efforts	Clinical, financial networking

Choosing a Future

Today's physicians are in transition. Hampered with increasing demands of patients and healthcare systems, physicians are under pressure to perform optimally. Tomorrow's physicians will need to reassemble old medical models and create new models. Either they'll play "poor me," working to treat people while medical business systems plot their passive future, or they'll have to work to treat people while they develop high-stakes partnerships with all the stakeholders involved in the creation and execution of healthcare delivery.

The change process can be positive. America is not only different from what it has been, it will never again be what it was, and neither will medicine. Considering what has changed since Fleming introduced us to antibiotics in the 1940s, greater cultural changes will lead either to a nihilistic society or one in which people values and honor each other. Focus groups were asked to turn analytical eyes to the future of organizational decision-making and power.

The Org Chart. Most physicians dislike direct lines of reporting to a supervisor. Most believe that automatically they have a dotted line to everyone and that they can practice medicine unsupervised. A nephrologist speaks his mind:

You have the brightest, most talented people at the front line. So if you were to design this as a traditional organizational chart you would find your brightest, most talented, most energetic people at the bottom of the org chart. But physicians don't know that. You know it's interesting to think of all the times you've approached organizational change and one of the first things people do is say, Well, let's see the org chart. Well, physicians don't really have that or else they can say, 'I am the org chart.' Physicians have to be more collaborative. As sole decision makers in healthcare, physicians need to change. I think they have to embrace the concept of using their skills to educate their patients to the extent possible to make the best long-term informed decision.

Vision. A physician recently promoted to the ranks of physician executive wrote:

Other people choose to be led by us because you represent something to them that they want to associate with. We must have and articulate a vision as a leader. People must buy into that vision. We need to demonstrate that vision. My passion is quality improvement and I feel there is a future for that. I think that aggregate data and working at quality across the spectrum of ambulatory and inpatient will be meaningful, and also meaningful to patients, employers and insurers. They will be able to

> demonstrate as physicians that they are as good or better at their job than anyone else. We lead by example and by what we stand for.

Another respondent said:

> A major challenge in leading physicians is the lack of a common goal within medicine. Medicine has been based on the physician/patient relationship and the goals were connected to the relationship and the outcome of the particular problem.

Integration. There was some broad discussion about the challenge of dealing with physicians who have practiced in different environments. Some have been in groups where they discussed how to practice better. Others have been independent and want to practice medicine as they always have. The challenge lies in integrating the two groups.

Physician backgrounds. Physicians and managers differ in how they've been trained: Physicians are used to working one-on-one; managers are used to working in a group setting. It's hard to get either to cross the line into the other's realm. A family physician said:

> For physicians there is ready gratification knowing at the end of the day that you've accomplished something. With management, it can take months to get the gratification that you deserve. The mind-sets are so different. The only way that will ever be resolved is if, at the very moment physicians and administrators begin their training; they learn to understand each other. By that I mean they have to understand how different both kinds of training have been, and the training itself has to be modified so they can work together and communicate.

Listening skills. A physician executive who serves in an administrative capacity 75% of the time and the balance in the clinic, pointed to the skill necessary for leadership:

> The most important thing you can do in leading physicians is to listen. It would be best to have administrators who have had experience practicing medicine. Most physicians still want to help people, but many today want a high quality of life in return. The greatest block to overcome in changing physicians' thinking or behavior is forgetting your own ego. We need to be firm, consistent, have standards, and live by them, and do it with compassion, allowing physicians to maintain their dignity.

Unraveling and Re-Birth

Leading and Managing. An orthopedic surgeon wrote:

> Physicians need to accept the mission of working together. They need to have a sense of community among themselves. We need physicians to lead physicians. We have to stay motivated about measuring outcomes and data evaluation. We need to keep up in order to keep the physicians we lead motivated about all of the changes that are going on.

Another person said:

> It's important to get physicians involved in managing. Treat physicians as professionals and with the respect they deserve. If you can work from the perspective of what's best for the patient in most issues, then the conflict would be lessened. Then everyone is trying to reach the same goal. Physicians and managers have the same thought processes in dealing with problems. If physicians could be trained to transfer the way they think clinically to the way they think managerially and understand the parallels, it would help a lot.

Another: "Physicians should not be managed by outside organizations, but rather they should be empowered by corporate medicine."

And another: "We need to get them to work together as a team. Also, to look at the patient as a whole person, not just a sum of various parts—an OB/GYN part, an internist part."

There was consensus that physicians usually are strong people with strong opinions who protect their turf. To lead them, individuals must be respected first, have high integrity, and be recognized in their fields. A hematologist in a focus group said:

> Doctors used to own patients, a patient was his *patient. That is not true anymore. Now the only owner is the insurance company and it is concerned only with the bottom line and sending the patients where it is the cheapest, not necessarily to the best doctor for that patient.

A psychiatrist addressing the medical society serves as a board member in a large metropolitan clinic:

> We need to get the leadership of medicine back in the hands of doctors. Business people are ill equipped to lead in this profession. A doctor knows his patients, but someone sitting

Power and Leadership

> *behind a computer in a big building somewhere is telling him/her what he or she needs to do for that patient. It's very frustrating. Doctors are angry---not happy—and it's not about their lower salary; it's because they have no decision-making power. A happy doctor has happy patients. We can't forget that.*

This declaration came from a soon to be retired physician in otorhinolaryngology:

> *Leaders need to have their values in place: honesty, integrity, and genuine caring for people. It is also a challenge to find physicians who are good and place the care of patients first and economic reward second.*

A clinical pathologist received hoots and cheers following the observation that:

> *Leading physicians is like herding cats. Physicians are hardworking, independent spirits, bright people, who tend to have an entrepreneurial spirit. It is very hard to lead this kind of group. You must have patience, respect, and be held in high regard by your peers. Leadership skills can be learned, but if you don't have the respect of your peers, you'll never be a good physician executive.*

Cats Stranded in a Blizzard

If leading physicians is like herding cats, imagine a group of healthcare leaders huddled together in a five-year blizzard. This group of stranded healthcare movers and shakers includes a medical school dean, the CEO of a hospital, the administrator of a clinic, the medical director of a long term care facility, the president of a leading university, the chief financial officer of a bank, a proponent for alternative medicine, a healthcare consultant, a nurse, an insurance representative, and the COO of an HMO.

Some of us have known and lived through terrible winter blizzards: The wind howls around corners, under the eaves and through the cracks; it's cold and dark because the electricity failed when the poles and lines broke. TV and radio are useless; batteries in cars and flashlights die; roads are impassable, even if you can get out of the driveway. Cars are stuck, more and more people get stranded, and our machines become irrelevant. Life becomes elementary.

The group trapped in today's healthcare blizzard and associated paralysis is a strange extended family of marginally acquainted

Unraveling and Re-Birth

members who have been meeting out of a sense of duty, guilt, obligation, and politeness. They intended a brief meeting, but now they are stuck with each other, and they must deal with questions, dilemmas, dislikes, discouragements, and physical and mental difficulties. Healthcare organizations—hospitals, HMOs, clinics, insurance companies, providers—are each as unique as family members, as are the occupational segments within them. Given that healthcare is stuck in this kind of stressed situation, throwing us back into some elementary problems, we raise the following elementary questions in an effort to find some common ground for moving ahead:

- How will we live together?
- What kinds of breakdowns are possible? Social dislocation, joblessness, communication blackouts, family isolation?
- How vital will be the values of trust, patience, thrift, selflessness, and reliability?
- What about norms for living and working together?
- And teamwork?
- When will the blizzard end? When will the weather change? And what's next? Tornado? Hurricane? Flood? Sunny springtime? Hot summer?
- Will the group have a new model for living and working together?
- Will everyone be treated and respected as an equal partner?
- Will the group create and agree on an agenda, a contract that leads to a new model?
- Will the agenda for this consortium be fluid, fertile, and financial?
- What would cause anyone to leave the group and walk out into the Whiteout blizzard?
- Why will anyone stay?

The consortium in the blizzard represents influential and powerful players in the development and maintenance of healthcare models and best practices. As a family they will need to deal with their differences, celebrate the fact that new ideas can emerge from old practices and biases, and that the birth of a new paradigm of working together will be accompanied by both pain and rejoicing. The new paradigm for work is in progress. Because of the unraveling of healthcare and changing medical education, medical students and practicing physicians are negotiating a new future. The players sometimes are friends, sometimes adversaries, sometimes colleagues, and sometimes unknown to each other. There are powerful leaders among them, some waiting to swing into action, others waiting to be trained. Leadership models can help.

You may be familiar with Max DePree's book *Leadership Jazz*. CEO of Herman Miller and leading thinker on leadership, DePree very persuasively likens the art of leading to the art of jazz. One leadership model we'll look at comes from the realm of jazz. I believe it is adapted to the management of organizational environments and demands of the future. I've structured this "Jazz Band" model of leadership on the basis of my own experience playing in a jazz band.

Another model considered here is the "Symphony Orchestra" model. You can pick and choose from the model's concepts and behaviors those that best fit your philosophical persuasions and the needs of the organization you serve. You can modify them, improvising around your own ideas. Your talents in diagnosing problems and in handling ambiguities, together with developmental models that fit your style, preferences, and leadership situations, can help you to lead with grace and imagination.

Jazz Band Model

The present and future situations in healthcare call for the imagination and energies of its participants in the face of ongoing change and uncertainty. Individual contributions to the problem solving and decision-making within and among organizations must be solicited and rewarded. Creativity is needed on all fronts. Organizations have to learn to recognize, accept, and channel that creativity through flexible structures and agile work processes. The jazz band model addresses these needs. It:

- Brings the gifts of individuals to the unpredictability of the future
- Demands high-quality individual performance within the context of a group
- Expects creativity within the parameters of established rhythms, structures
- Draws out the best in all (musicians) members of the medical team

- **Bringing the gifts of individuals to the unpredictability of the future.** With quality management goals and processes that facilitate individuals' good work, leaders can reshape the organizational structures and environments. They can create and address new visions, enlisting the best work that people can bring to their professions.

- **Demanding high-quality individual performance within the context of a group.** An executive cannot run a clinic or hospital in isolation. A physician alone cannot operate the functions of even a very small office and maintain the intellectual or emotional balance he/she needs to care for patients well. The group, the medical team, must know the patient, diagnose the presenting problem together with related problems, determine the options for treatment and care together with the appropriate team members qualified to provide it. Addressing the whole patient, they have to communicate options clearly and honestly to that person, the family members or caregivers, receive approval for the options chosen by the patient or guardians, and follow through with treatment.

- **Expecting creativity within the parameters of established rhythms, structures.** In non-life threatening situations, there may be a dozen best ways to provide treatment. The rhythm in the context determines the tune played. One patient may be best served by rhythm and blues while another prefers country western. One treatment process does not serve all.

- **Drawing out the best in all (musicians) members of the medical team.** What in your environment prompts you to do your best work, to go beyond what is expected, to stretch yourself in order to delight others? In a jazz ensemble each person is free to set standards and exceed them, to experience other members' work as they exceed the highest standards possible. In the presence of achievers whose desire is to be the best and do the best, a person is motivated to do and be the same. When things are out of tune, winners look for solutions while losers make excuses.

Consider:
- Who is the leader and how is the leader chosen?
- What rewards are necessary or critical for the players?
- Are guidelines necessary for peak performance?
- If so, who develops them?
- When does a jazz band become professional?

Power and Leadership

Symphony Orchestra Model

The jazz band operates differently from the symphony orchestra, which provides another model. The Symphony Orchestra model:

- Follows a score written by the patient
- Utilizes the talents of members under the conductor/physician's direction
- Acts within timing and rhythm determined by circumstances critical to outcome

- **Following a score written by the patient.** "If you want to know how the patient is, don't ask the doctor, ask the patient," advises an ancient Yiddish proverb. The patient writes the score for the medical symphony.

- **Utilizing the talents of members under the conductor/physician's direction.** The physician serves as player/conductor. While the symphony's teamwork follows a script, there is some artistic latitude for performance; still, it is the conductor who shapes that art, not the individual players. The physician is the key person, particularly in life-threatening medical interventions; a physician need not do everything any more than a conductor needs to play every instrument. A conductor needs to know the total score while individual players must be aware of a single part. Medical conductors need to know the players, the score, and the appropriate timing and procedure.

- **Acting within timing and rhythm determined by circumstances critical to the outcome.** The timing and rhythm of interactions are largely determined by circumstances critical to the outcome, by the score itself. Life- threatening situations demand planning, attentive listening, knowledgeable and competent workers, precise and synchronized action, and the ability to swap one procedure for another in the event of a surprise or crisis. The patient's heartbeat is the beat.

Consider:

- Who auditions the players?
- Does the conductor audition each section player?
- Does a violinist audition other violinists?
- Who decides who plays first violin and second violin?

Unraveling and Re-Birth

- What motivators are critical to maintaining group collaboration?
- What reward system would be satisfactory to all players?

Who establishes the rules/guidelines? Who enforces the rules/guidelines?

All That Jazz

I have played in several jazz bands and orchestras. I've learned that there are bands and there are bands, orchestras and orchestras. My first jazz band experience was when my twin brother and I were 15. I played the piano and he the trombone. We were five players working together with uneven talent, immense enthusiasm, and untested experience. Our first problem was leadership. Someone suggested that we take turns. We couldn't agree how to do it. Finally we threw our names in a cap and asked the new sax player to pull out the name of our leader for the next semester. My name was pulled. Now what?

As the leader of a nameless, mediocre, rag-tag jazz band, I followed the advice of our father, a general contractor. I asked for volunteers to be librarian, rehearsal scheduler, chair arranger, and contact person. Our father knew very little about music and a lot about organizing people. It worked. I became the chief "nodder." In a jazz band, the players take turns running through the melody while others support that person with secondary lines, rhythmic balance, and bold inventions. It was fun, especially when we knew what we were doing. I nodded to each player when I determined that they had run out of creativity or breath or both, and indicated who would be next.

All we had in common was the "cheat sheet." The cheat sheet is a record of the melody and the supporting chords. In the jazz group, each person is free to develop and embellish the melodic line within the constraints of the chord construction. If the cheat sheet indicates that the first four measures are in the key of F, all members play in the key of F. At this point there is no room for deviation of any kind. When all players have done their "shtick," the leader says, "Four more bars in F and finish," or signals non-verbally when the piece is to end. At the end of the piece, the leader waves a hand or finger and the group concludes the piece together decisively.

The jazz band leadership model can work for primary care physicians. The leader is asked to understand the system, the situation, and the strategy of care. The medical team members are ready for essentially non-emergency interventions.

Power and Leadership

Leadership Situations

Physicians face different types of situations, the outcomes of which may not be known. They enter into unpredictable futures in the short and long terms. The Jazz Band model, the Symphony Orchestra model, or any other model is more functional in some situations than in others. For instance, longer-term management strategies and non-emergency medical situations might best apply the jazz band approach. Crisis situations need crisis plans and crisis scripts at the ready, the symphony approach. Different configurations suggest what kind of leadership best fits treatment strategies:

Four distinct and yet interrelated functions point out the need for and differences between roles and responsibilities. They are: (1) Painful situations; (2) Life Threatening Situations; (3) Annual Check Up; and (4) Specialized Team.

Painful situation	**Life threatening situation**
Generalists Optional procedures Common beat w/ solos Supporting team All players equal Coordinator	Specialized team Exacting procedures Common score Section leaders Single group leader
Annual check-up	**Specialized team**
Generalists Basic procedures Steady beat: no solos All players equal	Optional procedures Need determines score Group leaders Shared leadership

Painful situation. This situation is not life threatening. It is generally reserved for medical generalists, the primary care or family physician. Optional procedures are available for broken bones and fractures. The staff is well informed about common procedures and can shift easily from one procedure to another, depending on the needs of the patient. The medical team is supportive and moves easily from one patient to another. All players are equal and the physician serves as coordinator. The jazz band model applies.

Annual check-up. As with some popular melodies, this model represents basic, generic medicine. Generalists are trained to handle the common cold and infections. Basic procedures rule the process as in playing a brass or reed instrument. There are just so many ways to hold a trumpet and make it sound like a thing of beauty. The staff plays a steady beat. There are no solos. All players are equal and the physician serves as coordinator. The jazz band model is for the non-specialist, whereas the orchestra model is for the specialist involved in emergency, potentially life-threatening interventions.

Life-threatening situation. Suppose that the following communication was analogous to activity described in an operating room where there is redundancy, back-up personnel, and stand-by equipment in case of electrical or mechanical failures. Suppose further that it's you on the operating table. "For considerable periods the four oboe players had nothing to do. The number should be reduced and the work spread more evenly over the whole of the concert, thus eliminating peaks of activity. All the 12 violins were playing identical notes; this seems to be unnecessary duplication. The staff of this section should be cut drastically. No useful purpose is served by repeating on the horns a passage that has already been handled by the strings. It is estimated that if all redundant passages were eliminated the whole concert time of two hours could be reduced to 20 minutes and there would be no need for an interval."

Do you want to eliminate fail-safe procedures? Do you want everyone to be in charge, or no one? It would cost less if we did away with excess people and equipment and hired an inexperienced medical student to direct the staff.

The surgeon in the operating room must be in control of the processes and procedures. While s/he cannot complete any procedure in isolation, direction must be given to each team member who must also have the power to initiate and complete all procedures within their specific responsibility. Autocratic and participatory elements are both part of the leadership in the operating room.

The physician leadership orchestra model is for life-threatening situations. The patient writes the script and score.

Power and Leadership

Individual players have the opportunity to practice their parts before ever sitting with their section or the entire orchestra. The physician conducts the players, every section, to play their portion of the score competently or better.

Specialized team. Brain or heart surgery requires that each player in the operating room knows what to do, when to do it, and how to respond when the patient changes the tune. The surgeon holds the baton with confidence and skill. The surgical team must act in concert if the outcome, the total production effect, is successful. Well-trained players know the rhythm of the procedures and can do their work, play their part, effortlessly.

Music and Leadership

Musical works are as distinct, diverse, and unique as are the projects of one's medical practice. An effective physician leader, utilizing the jazz band, orchestra, or other leadership model, recognizes that most people:

- Can handle unvarnished facts about themselves or their organization
- Want to "own" a part of their organization
- Want to be treated as partners and have a voice in developing their organization
- Want to know about all future probabilities and possibilities
- Want to know how they are doing
- Want to contribute to the success of any venture

Teamwork and Trust

What can physician leaders do when, in their teams or their organization, trust fails, suspicion reigns, and cooperation turns into individual rivalries? Doctors know that treatment without diagnosis is malpractice. In the same way, treatment of a toxic group or organization without first conducting a credible assessment of its problems and strengths is counterproductive. Leaders can begin an assessment process by asking some basic questions associated with trust:

- Which norms, values, or other drivers create suspicion?
- Is distrust a result of failure to achieve results?

- Does distrust arise from organizational structures, individuals, policies, and/or procedures?
- Do key players have a history of questionable integrity?
- Is distrust based on people's failure to demonstrate empathy and concern?

The English word "trust" is related to the German word "trost," which means *"comfort."* We violate the so-called "comfort zones" of others when we break our promises, behave erratically, contradict our stated values, use empathy as a bargaining chip, and so on. Where there is personal discomfort of this nature, there are also blighted hope and energy, cynicism and trepidation.

Physicians are eminently qualified to diagnose medical difficulty and can transfer their diagnostic skills to assess basic moods in organizations. Physician leaders can generate more comfort and trust when they deal with the whole person and the whole system.

Trust among individuals empowers and liberates the mind and spirit of each. Trust gives license to think new thoughts, create new models of organization. In order to manage in an age of uncertainty, we must trust our colleagues and ourselves in the creative process. Stability and uncertainty are zones of reality and opportunity brought together in the leadership model known as "Zones of Leadership."

Seven Zones For Leadership

The "**Seven Zones For Leadership**" model developed by Robert W. Terry addresses the seven zones in which a leader has the opportunity to face the stability of the past and the uncertainty of the future in ways that respect both.

Each zone for leadership functions within a time frame – past to future and a context – from stability to chaos. Everyday, the world comes at us in many ways. At times, it is fixable and knowable, other times it is complex and vibrant and other times it is unknowable and unfixable. Leadership differs, depending on the world that comes at us. And, all action occurs in the present. We can look backward and forward, from what is happening now.

Let us look at these different world and time frames and figure out what leadership in the medical field really requires.

Power and Leadership

1. Stewardship (Preserve the best; own the rest)

Sacred history. The physician is expected to guard that history on behalf of the patient, to treat it with respect, and to insure its accuracy. The physician leader asks, "What do we preserve and what do we let go of?" The metaphor guiding this zone is: life is a gift (both wanted and unwanted). Memory is the principle anchor. There is a willingness to face hard truths and a commitment to preserve the best.

2. Expert Task Mastery (Excel at your skills: ignore the frills)

The physician has a set of competencies to address specific medical needs. A broken bone is set by the physician with the expertise to do so. The core competencies required are technical. The physician leader shares expertise and trains others to become experts, matching the right people with the right jobs, doing the right tasks at the right time. Efficiency and reliability are hallmarks of this zone.

3a. System Architect (Connect the dots; downplay the spots)

The family is a system of relationships bound together by physical, emotional, and spiritual needs and values. The physician understands the family system and maintains a relationship by scheduling and performing such services as the annual check-up of its members. The physician also understands positional authority and executive control. Physician leaders assess what infrastructures are needed for the organizational foundation and it involved the mastering of systems thinking. Teams and communication and linkages are critical. Practically, it means that leaders are to connect the dots and downplay the spots. Need assessments are usually utilized to gain information about the DNA of the organization.

3b. System Guidance (Buy into the team; don't separate and scream)

The patient, in concert with trusted medical professionals, sets health goals that are congruent with family (system) values. This is where the physician provided a deep sense of belonging to and identity with the organization and the patient. This requires emotional intelligence, team building, ethical awareness, and a sense of core and shared values. The metaphor for this zone is that life is a body, a living system.

4. Political Engagement (Share the power; get down from the tower)

Differences occur between physicians and physicians, between physicians and patients. A leader is expected to make available other points of view, such as a second opinion, when there is a question or disagreement regarding the diagnosis or treatment. A leader will regard differences as an opportunity for continuing dialogue and relationship building. Shared power, getting down from the tower, and participation are critical to this zone. The metaphor guiding this zone: life is conflict between ups vs. downs. Downs know a lot and that needs to be revealed. Staff participates. Truth is in the workers: reveal it. Speak up! Those at the top still hold veto power. The mission is engagement. The core competencies required are conflict negotiation skills and assessing who are the buffalos in the organization.

5a. Future Shape (Avoid deflection)

Leadership is owned shared vision. Leadership engages in futuring, focusing on the destination of the trip. Through participatory methods, the preferred future is created and plans devised to achieve it.

5b. Future Watch (Anticipating the future)

The leader will lay aside all thoughts of credit, power, and institutional correctness and bring together everyone involved in the development of healthcare to scan future possibilities of delivery, technology, and system appropriateness, and the related redeployment of resources. Leadership addresses a world that is unknown, yet able to be anticipated. Scanning, futuring focusing less on the destination and more on the trip; scenario writing, shifting from market share to opportunity share dominate this zone. The metaphor guiding this zone: life is a journey, less destination, more the trip. Core competencies required are pattern recognition, scanning, framing, metaphorical thinking and new insight generation.

6. Creating Meaning (Cope with fear: leadership is discerning meaning in permanent white water)

The leader will invite others to assume the roles of the artist and philosopher, asking individuals and groups to address questions of purpose and vision, living in the midst of chaos. Events occur that were not anticipated, not on anyone's radarscope. "Permanent white water" is ever-present requiring process wisdom and improvisational skills. No one is in charge. Together, people co-create the means with no certainty of the outcome. Fear is rampant as people try to make meaning out of events that do not readily yield to sense making. Core competencies required: process wisdom, courage, improvisation, drama, framing, humor, and playfulness.

7. Serving the Promise (Serve the best and face the rest)

The leader will challenge everyone to isolate every paradox that either inhibits or promotes authenticity in individuals and systems. The outcome is self-knowledge in the face of uncertainty and chaos. The adept physician is ready to deal with surprises and all realities that are unknowable. Core competencies required: deep self-awareness, adept wisdom, listening to the stirrings, mapping complex issues, polarity and paradoxical thinking.

The seven zones serve as a bridge for the leader over time. The center of the bridge is political engagement and future watch. To look back is to manage the past. To look ahead is to lead by laying aside the baggage, customs, rules, and correctness of the past. The paradigm shifts in the following illustration are observed from a position on the center of the bridge. In many cases, the physician leader must manage the past, exert expert skill, understand human and mechanical systems, and engage in human and scientific dialogue. The leadership required of physician leaders assumes an ongoing adaptability and a comfort with ambiguity.

Given the reluctance of physicians to manage anything together with the reluctance of executive/managers to manage physicians, it is critical that everyone engage in a serious conversation regarding the paradigm shifts that have already occurred and which some refuse to acknowledge.

Paradigm Shifts In HealthCare

FROM	TO
1. Primary focus on physician	Primary focus on patients and partnerships
2. Teaching medical students	Creating a learning environment
3. Individual focus	Team focus
4. Discrete disciplines	Inter-disciplinary
5. Isolated specialties	Integrated practices
6. Discipline-based practice	Wellness/illness prevention-based practice
7. Homogenous clinical staff (all specialists, all primary care, etc.)	Diverse clinical staff (disciplines integrated)
8. Academic-based and reputation-based medicine	Community-based and evidence-based healthcare
9. Fee for service	Performance-based compensation
10. Limited or lack of performance review	Regular review/measurement by peers/patients
11. Innovation based on individual initiative	Innovation encouraged system-wide; mistakes basis of critical learning

© Personnel Decisions International: Author: Warren M. Hoffman (Adapted)

> "Status quo.
> Latin for the mess we're in."
>
> -Jeve Moorman

Chapter 7even

Teams
and
Multi-Disciplinary Decision Making

It took only one year for the same people to go from first to worst. Incredible! A major league baseball team (Minnesota Twins) celebrated a world championship. A group of wannabes became the idols of millions. They were the best in the world. A couple dozen men of different colors, ethnic backgrounds, sizes, and languages were a team. Some were rookies, others were seasoned men of summer. They believed in each other, provided unbridled encouragement and support, put individual goals behind the team goal—nothing less than the world championship—and they got it.

A year later, their success is a shadow. Some individuals elevated their nose, pushed out their chests, and said, "I want more money. I'm the one who got us to the big game. I'm most important." The newspapers have a field day over the bickering, rivalries, back-stabbing, posturing. And, then, last place in the division: from first to worst.

Look at your medical team. MD, RN, LPN, PA—you can add to the list. What is the glue that holds you all together? Who holds you together? What are your common goals? Are you a jazz band or an orchestra? Are you a team or a group? Can your team or group exhibit adept decision-making? Can you be a band when appropriate, or an orchestra when necessary? Do you have non-performers, slackers, or members who play a different tune? Are all pulling their own weight? Can the group tolerate close scrutiny? The questions are those of people who value, and who are involved in, serious teamwork. To independent, autonomous contributors these are bothersome questions. Why should an individual contributor take time to answer them?

The simple, glib answer quickly becomes complex. First, many Americans are rugged individualists, right? They are proud to be self-reliant and to do what has to be done. The immigrant, the pioneer, and the Wild West live somewhere in our brains, inspiring our souls. Metaphorically, even the most gentle among us has to buy a horse, to ride with other rugged individualists to capture the bad guys, or herd the cattle, or settle the land. The myth receives more credence that reality warrants. It makes for good novels, not good medicine.

Teams and Decision-Making

Team or group?

Groups are not teams. So what is the difference between them? One set of distinctions indicates that, whereas a group is characterized by 1) *mutual interaction* and 2) *reciprocal influence*, a team has four identifying characteristics: 1) *strong sense of identification*, 2) *common goals*, 3) *task interdependence*, 4) *specialized roles*. A team has clear goals and have to work together to accomplish them in a specified time frame. A group has broad goals; they do not work together often and do not have a tight time frame. We call them 'executives'.

Dr. Bonnie Dunbar, an astronaut, wrote during her flight in 1992:

> *So, what does being "part of the team" mean? It doesn't always mean being the smartest or the fastest. It does mean recognizing the big picture goal and the contribution that each individual brings to the whole. It may not mean being the life of the party, but it does mean being able to get along with people and to tread a fine line . . . knowing when to compromise and knowing when to stand firm. And, in an organization such as ours with competitive individuals used to being on top of the hill, it means knowing when to be a Chief and when to be an Indian. In the astronaut office, mission specialists rotate through technical jobs and different responsibilities during flights. Sometimes they are Indians instead of Chiefs. Those who perform best and appear to be well regarded can do each equally well.*

Bonnie grew up on a farm where she was required to have some skills to perform very special tasks and other skills to be a generalist. On the farm she learned how and when to be a leader and when to be a follower.

Orms: Forming, Storming, Norming, and Performing

What have you learned about your participation in groups and in teams? What else do you need to know or learn? Raise your eyebrow if you are familiar with the concepts of forming, storming, norming and performing. For purposes of review, let's hum a few bars about each of these "orms."

Forming. Groups arise. Teams form. Teams are formed around a common purpose or goal. The members of the team often are chosen or

Unraveling and Re-Birth

volunteer because of their specific skills. Polite conversation, superficial sharing, and low trust usually punctuate their formation stage.

Storming. This stage is when differences emerge, when the negative stuff surfaces those individuals felt during forming. First impressions are challenged. Values are challenged. Places and spaces and faces are given names and characteristics. Alliances or cliques are built or torn down. Leadership is tested.

Norming. This is the stage when the culture of the team is defined and refined, when it's determined how the team will live and work together. It's the rule stage in which what is and is not acceptable finds definition and codification, and common goals and clearer roles are defined.

Performing. This is the ideal stage. The team has met, fought, bargained, and rolls up its sleeves and does the work. The group is now a team. Interdependence and collaboration reign.

Physician leaders who expect the group to meet-and-do or form-and-perform immediately are naive. It doesn't happen that way. No stage can be skipped. High performance teams are successful in various stages and on multiple levels: that of the organization the team serves, that of the team itself, and that of individual team members. According to *TeamWise* (the Team Success Model developed by PDI to build stronger organizations), the *impact* of an organization, its teams, and their members is driven by six critical factors:

Capabilities	Practices
Clarity	Power
Participation	Commitment

Impact: *The organization meets and exceeds its strategic goals. Teams make a significant contribution to the success of customers, team members, and the organization. Individuals achieve personal and professional goals.*

Capabilities	Power
The organization ensures teams have the resources to succeed. Teams have the right mix of talents. Individuals have the right skills and experience.	The organization holds teams accountable. Teams know their authority and can overcome obstacles. Individuals have confidence in their ability to succeed.

Teams and Decision-Making

Practices	Participation
The organization's policies and practices support and reward teams and teamwork. Teams own, manage, and continuously improve their processes. Individuals' work styles and behaviors support the work of the team.	The organization fosters cooperation among teams. Teams work effectively and create a positive team environment. Individuals contribute fully and encourage each other.
Clarity	**Commitment**
The organization has a clear mission and strategies. Teams have clear charters, goals, and measures for success. Individuals understand their roles and contributions.	The organization believes teams make a difference. Teams believe their work is valuable. Individuals are dedicated to the work of the team.

© *TeamWise* Personnel Decisions International

Two physicians discuss their experience in working on multi-disciplinary teams:
"To my surprise, my participation on several teams has been entertaining, a learning experience, and something I look forward to. I also try not to overextend myself."
"The multi-disciplinary teams that I have been a part of are dynamic. Communication is both formal and informal. You learn what to expect of each other in the ultimate goal of helping the patient."
"The multi-disciplinary team works if each person has the respect of all others on the team. As with team athletics, everyone has to work together or the sessions will fail. No one in the group must feel superior to any other. All ideas must be explored."

Benne and Sheats have outlined a series of work activities called role differentiations. Teams and groups assume informal and formal roles that can work in task-oriented settings, in building and maintenance, and in personal, self-satisfying roles.

Role Name	Task-Oriented roles: behaviors directed toward accomplishing the group's objectives, primarily through contributing to the problem-solving process
Initiator	Proposes tasks, goals, or actions; defines group problems; suggests work procedures

Informer	Offers facts, gives expression of feelings, gives opinions
Information seeker	Asks for opinions, facts, or interpretations
Clarifier	Interprets ideas or suggestions, defines terms, clarifies issues before the group
Summarizer or coordinator	Pulls together related ideas, restates suggestions, offers a decision or conclusion for group to consider
Reality tester	Makes a critical analysis of an idea, tests an idea against some data to see if the idea will work
Procedural technician	Records suggestions, distributes materials
Energizer	Attempts to increase the quality and quantity of task behavior
Elaborator	Expands on suggestions, offers examples, restates positions, offers rationales
Consensus tester	Asks to see if a group is nearing a decision, sends up a trial balloon to test a possible conclusion
Building and maintenance roles:	Social-emotional behaviors aimed at helping the interpersonal functioning of group. Like the maintenance required to keep a car in good running condition, these behaviors are necessary to keep group members feeling good about the group and interacting effectively with one another.
Harmonizer	Attempts to reconcile disagreements, reduces tension, gets people to explore differences
Gatekeeper	Helps keep communication channels open, facilitates participation of others, suggests procedures that permit sharing remarks
Encourager	Friendly, warm, and responsive to others, indicates by facial expression or remark the acceptance of others' contributions
Compromiser	When own idea or status is involved in a conflict offers a compromise that yields status, admits error, modifies an interest of group cohesion or growth
Observer or commentator	Comments on and interprets group's internal process
Follower	Serves as audience, passively goes along with ideas of others

Teams and Decision-Making

Personal roles:	Intended to satisfy individual needs rather than contribute to goals or maintenance of group. Although some personal role behaviors do contribute to group's effectiveness, roles characteristic of this category are irrelevant to goals of group and not conducive to its functioning
Aggressor	Deflates others' status: attacks the group or its values, jokes in a barbed or semi-concealed way
Blocker	Disagrees and opposes beyond reason, resists stubbornly the group's wishes for personal reasons, uses hidden agenda to thwart movement of group
Dominator	Asserts authority or superiority to manipulate group or certain group members, interrupts contributions of others, controls by means of flattery or other forms of patronizing behavior
Prince or Princess	Makes a display of own lack of involvement, "abandons" the group while remaining with it physically, seeks recognition in ways not relevant to group task
Evader	Pursues special interests not related to tasks, stays off subject to avoid commitment, prevents group from facing up to controversy
Help seeker	Uses group to gain sympathy and solve personal problems unrelated to group's goal
Recognition seeker	Calls attention to self by boasting and referring to personal achievements, acts in appropriate ways to gain attention
Special-interest pleader	Speaks on behalf of represented group in order to cloak own prejudices or biases in a stereotype that fits own personal needs rather than goals of the current group

Multi-Disciplinary Decision Making

A decision is a step taken to make progress in solving, resolving, or dissolving problems. Collaborative decision-making within a multi-disciplinary environment is complex in that while some may wish to solve a problem, others may wish to ignore it or dissolve it. While the collaborative approach is more desirable than the autocratic approach, it is more time-consuming and requires everyone's more active listening and serious attention to all points of view.

Using the JAZZ model, described earlier, the healthcare team can make decisions in treating illness or disease. The Jazz model supports leadership without authority (as opposed to authority without leadership). All players are expected to contribute their expertise in a timely and appropriate way depending on the rhythm set by the patient's need. Since there are many acceptable treatments possible in non life- threatening situations, the team has more latitude for creativity. New ways of treating well-known illnesses are possible.

The team is not dependent on external permission or expectations to find new and more effective ways to bring about health. It can focus on the issues of the illness rather than on protocols. The team can get closer than any one person can to the patient's history, needs, reactive patterns, and pains. It's the team that brings focus, attention, and technology together, and may thereby invent better practices in the diagnosis and treatment.

Questions to Consider

The following questions serve as an audit for both individual team members and the group as a whole. If you are involved in a team or group problem-solving process, you might streamline their work by getting this information out before it begins its formal work and might otherwise have to spend collective time establishing such points.

- Who owns the problem? (Person, department, committee, organization)
- What information is available to begin formulating a decision?
- Is the problem(s) structured, organized, or diffuse?
- If a single person or a group made the decision, would others accept it? Reject it?
- Where are the landmines, traps, and roadblocks?
- What kind of decision is required?
- What is the timetable?

Once group work is underway, consider these questions: Is conflict preferred over a solution? A decision *not* to seek a solution is a decision to maintain the status quo and often that means an organizational conflict. Is the problem(s) linked with organizational goals, values? What if nothing is done? What are the options for treatment and potential benefits/problems, including doing nothing? What is the best decision? And does that decision involve the patient?

A variety of decisions must be made to solve, resolve, or dissolve the patient's problem(s), which may be described in terms of pain. Team members are expected to raise questions that eventually will lead to the multi-disciplinary decision-making process. The context

Teams and Decision-Making

will determine the kind of leadership required, and the patient will help to determine if the situation is life threatening or not.

- The **anesthetist** must ask: "Are all the backup systems in place?"
- The **nurses** must ask: "Have we covered all the details?"
- The **surgeon** must ask: "What else needs to happen to be ready? Any unfinished business with anyone? This patient is depending on us."
- The **operating room staff** must ask: "Are we ready for the unexpected?"
- The **nurse manager** must ask: "Who will step in if someone drops out physically?"
- The **administrator** must ask: "Is all the people work and paper work in order?"
- The **chaplain** must ask: "Is this person ready to deal with the emotional and spiritual trauma?"
- The **patient** must ask: "Do I understand what is happening to me and what this medical staff plans to do about it? How comfortable do I feel that I and they are doing the right things for me?"
- The **family** must ask: "What can we do to help? For what must we be ready?"
- The **team leader** (physician) must ask: "Have we considered everyone's perspective, including the patient's? Have we made the best decision under the circumstances?"

The Medical Team and Consensus

A medical team is usually organized around a specific purpose or need. Its team might work together for an hour, a month, or longer. The dimension of time and the makeup of the team are determined by the purpose or need. Team leaders can be assigned or chosen informally by the team members. The most effective teams are those with diverse perspectives, experiences, and competencies to bring to decision making and consensus building processes.
Consensus building takes time. Both a peril and an opportunity, it's often messy and noisy. Process can guide attempts at consensus building:
- *Defining* the problem(s). (When all parties agree on definition they go to next step.)
- *Generating* alternative problem-solving strategies and problem solutions.

- *Gathering* knowledge, information, perspectives.
- *Discussing*, with now informed dialog, the alternative solutions and their implications.
- *Reaching* agreement on which alternative to use.

At its best, multi-disciplinary decision-making can be enriching for physicians while complementing their skills. At its worst, it can take an inordinate amount of time and not even reach satisfying resolutions. It can be fragmented by poor communication among the decision makers. Adequate and informed discussion is necessary among team members.

Multi-disciplinary decision-making is becoming an essential part of rehabilitation and related medical specialties. It supports the unique contribution of all team member participants to given patient treatments and care. To patients, it remains a foreign concept until they experience its value firsthand.

A Peril. Physicians have a history of being decisive and are seldom celebrated for their patience. They are action and task-oriented. They have little experience with the dynamics of group process. Most physicians like to solve the problem alone, using the information available at the time. Physicians on the go and in a hurry often call the time-consuming process of consensus a waste of time. "I don't have time for this. I didn't go to medical school to sit in meetings. I'm here to cure patients." A principle peril for physicians involved in consensus building is impatience, compounded by sensitive issues of an ego claiming to know it all. Patients are not concerned about how a decision is made as long as it has a positive impact. Patients also can be impatient and want an immediate answer.

The Opportunity. If physicians want to discover or invent new ways to treat patients, or new ways to make things easier for staff and patients, they will connect the knowledge and experience of all participants in the process. Multi-disciplinary problem solving and decision making enhance that connection. One contributor to this book notes:

> *The basic idea could be terrific. If properly managed, it could be enriching for physicians and complement their skills. The multi-perspective is valuable and essential in some specialties like rehabilitation where all aspects need to be taken into account. There are too many decisions not to involve a group of experts. Ultimately, patients will receive better care with a*

Teams and Decision-Making

variety of unique contributions. If one expert is myopic, an experienced group can challenge intellectual and emotional biases. There is safety in numbers. The multi-disciplinary team can engage in target practice with new practices.

When nothing gets done. Nothing is *something*. To avoid nothingness in the decision-making process the team needs to clarify at the beginning what kind of decision is hoped for, what objective is sought.

Example: "We have several problems in the ER: our costs are out of line, our staffing is uneven, our supplies are either in short supply or overstocked, our documentation is seriously flawed. Where do we start?"

Put off: "Let's find out what other hospitals are doing first." or, "Form a task force to investigate."

Act dumb: "I don't understand. Say that another way? Get me more information so I can ask the right questions."

Sabotage: Destructive participants find ways to plant landmines and construct roadblocks, ways to say yes and mean no. "I really like that idea, but . . ." "I'll do the internal survey and find out how many people really want this." "We tried that last year, you know. We won't do well with consecutive failures, but if that's what you want . . ." "It would take *how much* time?"

Process observation and consultation. A designated process observer may take notes during the session and comment on what is happening without editorializing or passing judgments. The purpose of process observation is to ensure listening, accuracy in reporting group consensus and decision making, and the intellectual and emotional inclusion of all parties. Example:

> *Pat began the meeting 10 minutes after the stated start time. The secretary apologized for not having a printed agenda. Chris said that she was upset since this was the third meeting without a written agenda. Coffee was brought in after 20 minutes and we took about 10 minutes filling cups, and joking around after Harry spilled his coffee on Max's shoes. Jon noted that we seemed to be stalled and felt lost. No one responded. Sue went to the board and wrote, WE DON'T GET IT. It was quiet for a minute and then Chris suggested that we write out the agenda.*

Unraveling and Re-Birth

Process consultation begins after the process observation. The observer can be an internal consultant and say, "It looks like we have some unfinished business around the table. Chris might like to talk about his concerns. Jon might like to tell us how he feels and Sue could tell us what she meant by her statement on the board. If this is appropriate, any of you may respond."

Behind closed doors. Decisions made behind closed doors usually involve sensitive issues about the future of individuals or organizations. Recognizing that there are no perfect decisions, our better decisions are made when we have adequate data based on the input of all strategic thinkers and players. Our worst decisions are made in the spirit of revenge, anger, or unexamined discontent.

Model for Decision Making.

The following model addresses two critical factors: causes and outcomes. Each preference indicated has a specific goal supported by a desire to:

Compromise:
Use when individuals agree on expected outcomes, not on the relative outcomes.

Computation:
Use for efficiency when key individuals are certain about outcomes.

Inspiration:
Use to exercise strong hunches and achieve inspiration when there is disagreement about the consequences.

Judgment:
Use to make decisions in complex and uncertain situations to reach clear-cut objectives.

High		
	Compromise	**Computation**
	Goal is value, harmony	Goal is efficiency
Belief About		
Causation		
	Inspiration	**Judgment**

Teams and Decision-Making

Low	Goal is based on hunches, guesses, or intuition	Goal reached when preferences are clear and judgment is required to reach them
	Disagreement	**Agreement**

Case Study

The North Central Healthcare Alliance was created in 1997 as a result of four merging entities: Axel Insurance Company, Maxwell Hospital (for profit), St. Luke's General Hospital, and Community General Hospital (tertiary hospital). The chief executive officers of each entity were retained and remained essentially in their previous positions. G. Stanton Ellsworth, as the former CEO of Axel Insurance Company, is the chairman of the new organization. His principle concern is efficiency. Edward Helms is the CEO of St. Luke's. He values compromise. Community General's CEO is Ann Marie Clement, who values good judgment and clear-cut objectives. Pat Hanson is the CEO of Maxwell Hospital where decisions are intuition based.

Weekly executive meetings are designed to deal with financial and market issues. Other concerns may be discussed and are given less time and attention. After Several weeks it becomes clear to Helms and Hanson that the executive meetings lack good will and high energy. They decide to address their concerns at the next meeting of the executive group.

Pat takes the lead at the beginning of the meeting. "I'm concerned that we may not be on the same page. I'm also a bit anxious that we may not have dealt very well with how we make decisions together."

"I share your concern," Edward responds. "We look at numbers more than we look at each other. We need to decide what really counts. We're in healthcare business and healthcare is all about health and caring. I think we need to care about each other and I'd like to talk about it sometime. Maybe even now."

Ann Marie moves boldly into the conversation. "This is not our regular format for executive meetings, but I'm willing to have both of you present your facts and arguments in a white paper so we can more appropriately think about the issues. I don't think today is the day to do this."

Stanton continues to look at his financial report, shuffles his papers and says, "I'm ready to discuss the number-one item on the agenda, namely the capital fund reserve allocations. We can let the personnel people come in and talk to us later. Now, how do you suppose we can stabilize the reserve fund?"

Edward and Pat say nothing as they defer to Stanton, who continues to direct the discussion and then concludes the meeting as though they hadn't introduced their concerns. The issues of decision making and caring about what really counts go PLOP!

But... Meetings don't have to go badly. Problem solving and decision-making don't have to collapse in a puddle. When all the individuals on the team take responsibility for remaining conscious, and moreover attentive, as well as honest and committed to the process, group dynamics can build a positive momentum. Individuals on their own cannot change systems or entrenched structures - teams can.

One more true life story from a physician leader.

After failing repeatedly in my effort to evoke thoughtful conversation about our decision making process I finally decided to explore major and complex decisions we had made as a team. I selected three major decisions that were implemented with relative easy and three that were characterized by more than a few, myself included, as unmitigated disasters.

I couldn't get my leader colleagues to talk about it. It would get on meeting agendas but there was never time. Instead we talked about what Covey called things that are "important and urgent" and not things that were important and not urgent like our decision making process. My sense was that there was a lot of resistance around the use of a participative process out of fear that their preferred direction might not prevail. Essentially I saw it as a lack of trust of the staff know the truth and act wisely.

Failing any progress with my leader colleagues I made a presentation to our elected physician board of nine practicing physicians. It was scheduled as an educational session on leadership. I asked them it list recent major organizational decisions that went well

Teams and Decision-Making

in terms of implementation and to list decisions that were poorly received, poorly implemented or that generated revolt. Their list included, among others, the six examples I had generated. I then asked the group over an hour and a half to talk about the characteristics of the process for decision making in each case and to see if there was anything to learn. The conversation was animated and the conclusions seemed to have a lot of consensus.

1. First there needed to be a clearly articulated appropriate and generally understood process for making the decision in advance. This helped provide a process for information sharing and direction for those who needed to be heard and/or wished to be heard.
2. Open, honest and non-defensive information sharing on the part of leaders was essential to building trust.
3. Authentic listening: to all voices helped to create confidence and credibility and acceptance of the decision.
4. Doctors don't expect to always have their way. They do expect to be heard and for the process to be open and "fair".
5. Institutional recognition and memory about those who sacrificed in one decision would mean that the sacrifice would be remembered the next time there was need for sacrifice. This way there could be a sense of balanced distribution of the sacrifice.

I was delighted I got great feedback from the elected physician board The CEO and COO sat and silently observed.

*Back at the office the next day the COO and current CEO confronted me in the hall and said that my session was extremely frustrating for him. The CEO, hearing the comment, came out of his office and chimed in Dueck and I lust don t agree when **it** comes to decision making and walked away My heart sank, not because of the put down. Rather it sank because we would make no progress in our decision making in the future. For years the CEO and I had been kidding each other. I characterized his process as "ready, fire, aim" and he characterized my more participative process as "ready, aim, aim ,and aim . . ."The trouble was that the conversation never got any deeper than that. My thought was with the TV commercial that said "pay me now or pay me later". The incredible thing is this. Both the CEO and COO are wonderful human beings deeply dedicated to their work and doing the right thing. They would "climb any mountain and ford any stream" to help the organization. It seems this is true except for the willingness to* *look inside themselves. (my bias) The group had handed them a blueprint for more effective decision making and they couldn't even see it. From my perspective, they were blinded by fear.*

Now that I think about it the model that I said I had trouble picking up on might be relevant complex decisions require a different process than simple, cut and dried ones. We don't manage a cardiac arrest by committee."

What next? Creative wrestling with partnerships and polarities.

Teams and Decision-Making

> "It wasn't raining when Noah built the ark."
>
> -Howard Ruff

Chapter 8ight

Partnerships

Brian Campion, M.D., M.P.A.

As a practicing cardiologist, physician executive, and now a physician educator, I'm convinced that we must rethink every system and process that we call healthcare. The basic groups or stakeholders including patients, providers, payers, employees, governmental agencies, and insurers must participate in serious dialogue about systems and processes. We must have representatives from every group at the table. WE must engage in fresh dialogue where we seek common ground rather than seek dominance of one group over another. Physicians must take a special role in stimulating and sustaining this discussion because of their primary contract with the patient and the fact we are knowledgeable of the processes within the continuum of care which will need redesigning. To occupy this central position with the permission of the other stakeholders, the doctors must renounce self-interest and commit to the dictum that *"the needs of the patient come first."*

The welcome promise by managed care of better care at the same or lower cost was eagerly embraced by consumers, the government and employers. Government through its entitlement programs was bearing a disproportionate percentage of healthcare costs even as the national debt increased. Employers, many participating in the global marketplace, found their healthcare costs and hence their product costs higher than competitors from other nations. The remedy of the late 80s and early 90s for American business faced with similar problem had been to redesign processes of production to improve quality and at the same time lower cost. They saw managed care as a promise to take the same road as American manufacturing and service industries.

Until recently managed care was successful in slowing the growth of costs with no demonstrable adverse effect on quality. The effect on cost was brought about by reduction in hospital charges due

Partnerships

to shorter lengths of stay, reduction in physician salaries and shifting more cost to individual consumers. Consolidation of the hospital industry through mergers and acquisitions resulted in some savings. Shortened lengths of stay with more care provided in shorter periods by fewer people led to reduced costs but little redesign of care processes. These changes have recently raised questions of falling quality of care as suggested by studies documenting the high frequency of medical error in hospitals. Physicians have moved from their own practices into larger organizations where behaviors and salary can be better controlled. In short, we have moved from healthcare as a cottage industry to fewer, larger, organizations with a new culture and many dissatisfied employees and patients (customers).

Other practices which cause increased medical costs include:

- Failure to manage patient expectations of access to any desired care even as the population ages.
- Isolation of physicians in the decision-making process while care becomes more complex, malpractice suits rise and the physician is more financially at risk.
- Ignorance of caregivers regarding the real cost of ambulatory, emergency, and routine care.
- Ineffective training programs to make real changes in how caregivers are trained.
- Inappropriate use of and the rising cost of pharmaceuticals.

These and other root problems plus the fact that care is delivered by new healthcare organizations strongly indicates the need for redesign of the processes of care. The redesign of care must involve all stakeholders in a cooperative fashion to show no sign of starving care. Costs will continue to rise. The quality of care must rise even faster if the value of American healthcare is to be improved.

If the partnerships between and among all stakeholders are to thrive, the physician must be included and set aside real or potential arrogance and become an informed, servant of the redesign. American physicians find themselves in a new environment without their previous all powerful position and bereft of credible leadership. In short we are in turbulent seas without a compass and with no

Unraveling and Re-Birth

rudder on the healthcare ship. The compass in the past has always been the needs of the patient come first, and the rudder that steered the ship was a commitment to the standards of learned profession. Only if we reaffirm these tenants and empower physician leaders who can we sit at the table, and speak the language of modern healthcare, will we return to our traditional place of leadership.

What do we have in common?
That's the first question for every stakeholder.

The first assignment, then, is to wrestle with the process to determine what unites us. It is not a simple task.

"The tragedy of the commons" a tale in Jedidiah Purdue's book, "*For Common Things*" is informative and telling. Listen to his story.

"*My parents came to West Virginia in 1974, the year I was born. They meant to live with few needs, to raise as much of their own food ad do as much of their own work as possible, and to share what they could not do themselves with like-minded neighbors. As my father once said to me, they intended 'to pick out a small corner of the world and make it as sane as possible.' They chose a little more than a hundred acres, mostly steep, eroded pastures and second-growth oak woods, in the uneven bowl of a broad hollow. One side of the hollow was steep and wooded, the other gentler and cleared as meadow. At its back the bowl's lip lowered into a gap between two ridges. At the end of our property the hillsides drew into a narrow passage, where our creek leapt out into a waterfall, and our dirt road clung to the hillside.*
Our home is still there, and the land is unchanged."

Purdue go on to describe common education and neighborhood experiences where people shared things, even grazing land, daredevil carpentry, the woods and meadows, tools and ideas. The common land between neighbors was everyone's land and no one's land. It belonged to everyone. And what if one neighbor became greedy and claimed what belonged to everyone? What if someone did not agree to the value of sharing? What happened when trust eroded? What happened when people stopped listening to each other, even the children?

Partnerships

Where do we begin?

In the past physicians have been undisputed captains of the healthcare ship. With a reactive style and problem solving approach the doctor-captain has led the response to an identified disease. Recent experience has demonstrated that prevention also has a major role to play. Whether in prevention of disease itself or further episodes of an already established condition the members of the team are changing their focus. This new focus requires an expanded team of professionals cooperating to provide better care for each episode of illness and to prevent recurrence. This necessary teamwork mandates the formation of partnerships across a wide spectrum of providers and in various settings. The doctor's role remains central because the patient doctor bond must continue across the spectrum of care.

Essential to any partnership is significant commonality of values or systems of beliefs. For example, recent evidence would indicate that the sister operated Catholic hospitals and their physician medical staff have common values such as the patients needs come first and the desire to serve. At times what they value is different but the commonality of the values encourages excellent patient care. In other words a common set of values help structure a partnership strategy. The following values and objectives are submitted as discussion starters:

- Healthcare is for everyone.
- All partners to be treated with respect.
- The purpose of healthcare is to insure healthy individuals and communities.
- Differences are honored in the spirit of dialogue.
- Barriers to and the burdens of the partners are shared.
- Cost reduction follow quality of care.
- The pulse of the partnership will be taken regularly.

Why have past attempts at stakeholder dialogue been so unsuccessful? One answer would be that each group has brought their own thinly disguised self-interest to the table with little or no desire to compromise. Physicians have brought a profound knowledge of patient/provider relations and parochial economic self-interest as well as a history of being in charge. Administrators,

MBA's, MAA's have brought an understanding of finance and organizational structure without a clear understanding of the care of their business; patient/provider relationship. Patients continue to see healthcare as a right and steadfastly rebuff attempts to be made more accountable. Payers continue to lobby for short team gain over sustained results. The only question now is whether all stakeholders have failed sufficiently to adopt other strategies. Many experts feel that the quality of care is at stake so other strategies must be tried.

There seems to be general agreement that physicians can best influence patient's behavioral change whether it is in compliance to therapeutic regimes or stopping harmful behaviors such as smoking. Coupled with the previous referenced understanding of processes of care, the physician must be contributing member of the team of change. Unfortunately, physicians have little history of being partners with non-physicians, especially if they hold financial risk, as is the case today.

Despite the history of not working in teams physicians today find themselves in different circumstances. As noted above, doctors have increasingly become part of large organizations which over time will encourage more collaborative behavior. Secondly, in the age of specialization, no one physician has all the answers. Whether it be medical specialist, or allied health experts such as nurses or physical therapists, today's medical care increasingly is provided within organizations by teams of people. Physicians likely will play varying roles on that team, sometimes as leaders, but often as team members.

A necessary first step in partnering is to bring the stakeholders together for development of common ground. Beginning with the discussion of common values, clarified by what each stakeholder values, the potential partners should then come to agreement of mission, vision, and strategy. I have been party to this kind of effort and aware of the patience, good, will, respect, humility, and listening required to stay on track.

The redesign process must begin and end with...

- Desired outcomes
- Guiding principles and values
- Rules of engagement

Partnerships

- Measurement of processes and outcomes
- Alignment of incentives between all stakeholders

We are all aware that real change only comes when staying the same is not an option. Currently some stakes holders such as physicians and nurses are finding themselves in the untenable position of trying to live to their professional standards and providing cost effective care. Some patients such as the working poor and impoverished elderly are not able to afford needed care. Stuck with an increasing role of the health bill, government makes reimbursement cost which effect quality of care. Employees and insurers are poised to have their costs once again escalate. There are no easy answers so maybe now will be the time to form the partnerships that can bring better quality of care with the same or lower cost. It is possible but not in a system of winners and losers.

Old methods no longer work, the trust level between the public and the healthcare systems including providers have never been lower, the financial crisis is real and unabating, there is evidence that despite technological and pharmaceutical advances the quality of care is suffering and lastly healthcare is out of sync with industry and other essential parts of society. Desperate times call for desperate measures. Physicians, healthcare leaders and other stakeholders must put aside parochial interests and past grievances.

The goal here is attainable if and when all parties agree the status quo is untenable. A necessary first stop in partnering is to bring the stakeholders together for an understanding of common ground, creating an understanding of what is best for the whole. **Beginning with the discussion of common values, desired outcomes and governed by rules of engagement of measurement of processes and outcomes, real partners can then come to agreement regarding mission, vision and strategy.**

Unraveling and Re-Birth

Chapter Nine
Polarity and Paradox Re-Visited

A polarity is the possession or manifestation of two opposing attributes, tendencies or principles that are interdependent. They identify a relationship that is ongoing and raise issues that do not go away. A polarity is not an either/or decision, a continuum, a mystery or a compromise.

A colleague, Bob Terry, outlines a series of examples of polarities in his book, Seven Zones for Leadership:

> Part/Whole
> Dynamic/Form
> One/Many
> Unity/Diversity
> Individual/Team
> Reveal/Conceal
> Ends/Means
> Serious/Play
> Inside/Outside
> Stability/Change

These polarities get expressed in the following set of polarities within organizations:

Cost	And	Quality
Market Driven	And	Product Driven
Centralized	And	Decentralized
Innovation	And	Standardization
Autocratic	And	Participatory
Process Engineering	And	Product Engineering
Planning	And	Taking Action
Common Computer Systems	And	Custom Computer Systems

Source: Barry Johnson

A paradox is an absurdity, irony, contradiction, and inconsistency. Every part of a paradox is linked to itself and cannot exist apart from it. To separate one part of a paradox from itself it to pronounce paradoxical death. Examples of paradox include:

Polarity and Paradox

Night and Day
Woman and Man
Up and Down
In and Out
Left and Right
Light and Dark
Wet and Dry
Rich and Poor
Freedom and Bondage
Big and Small

Why address issues of polarities and paradoxes? They are real, ever present and will not go away.

- Traditional approaches offer false promise and hope – paradoxes persist.
- The dilemma of "white water." Change vs. huge bureaucracies.
- Push to simplify – try to avoid contradictions – quick fix.
- Rise of charismatic management gurus.
- The age of the cult company. Best practice – highly visible.
- Endless management proposals – the "re" age.
- Good intentions lead to unintended results.
- Opens question of spirituality in the work place.

Healthcare is currently in the grip of the polarity and paradox. Polarities can be managed; a paradox cannot. The quick-fix mentality results in many decisions being made to satisfy those who engage in *ready, fire, aim* behavior.

An example of operational polarity is with the physician who spends half time as a medical director, executive partner, or other titles indicating that s/he is not a full-time clinician. The physician-executive is an ambiguous anomaly, an abnormality in the medical setting that gets respect only when it's treated.

On the one hand, the administrators want to work with physicians who can speak the language of budgets, ratios, revenue projections, a language not based on 'unreality of Latin lingo' spoken by the pharmaceutical crowd.

On the other hand is the physician-clinical group who looks at the physician-executive as a traitor, one who has abandoned the purities of clinical work in favor of numbers, charts, and accountants. The physician-executive gets the silent treatment, and is dealt with on the basis of professional passive-aggressive interaction. What does that mean?

It means dishonesty.

When meeting with physicians, the physician-executive has the responsibility of explaining new procedures, new relationships with third party payers, customer expectations, and a host of administrative policies that directly impact the quality of healthcare deliver. The passive-aggressive listeners nod their heads in accent during the meeting and following the meeting criticizes the presenter, the presentation, the policies, procedures, and all physicians who become the 'suit'. So who wants to become a physician-executive?

And what about physicians who are department chairs? In clinics and hospitals where there are no direct reports, no supervisors or bosses, how does one lead a group of peers over whom s/he has no authority? What if there is an honest difference between cost and quality? What if the group is split? Who decides?

A physician in this dilemma faced with peers who would not and could not reach consensus, said, *We struggled in the spirit of good will until the good will ran thin. We were stuck. I am the so-called head of the group (32 docs of all ages). The older physicians refused to discuss any change. The younger ones were all for it. I'm in the middle of the age bracket (45). Any decision I made would anger half of the group. Here I am, the leader and I don't know how to lead. I'm stuck, too. It was like I was the president of the U.S. Senate and there was a tie vote. I'm not paid extra for this kind of grief. And so in the meeting, all eyes were on me. The silence was deafening. I had to gamble. I was in favor the change and knew that support would come from the younger physicians.*

I took a sheet of paper, scribbled a brief note in effect submitting my resignation as the managing partner, folded it and kept it until after I spoke to the entire group.

I support the change we're discussing which in effect will split the group. And, giving the paper to a person sitting next to me, said, I now submit my resignation and ask you to act on it. If you want me to continue, I will. If you want another person to assume this responsibility, I gladly accept your vote and will fully support the next partner.

I sat down and waited.
Nothing happened for what seemed like an eternity. I was likely no more than a minute. I was hoping someone would step up to the plate.
One of the older physicians (62), spoke first.
"I'm about ready to cash in. I'm working too hard and don't want more work. The change we're talking about will mean more work and I'm getting tired. I was selfish in my vote. If the change can mean that my work load can get lighter or remain the same, I'm for it. You young people have more stamina and need more money than I do. Twenty years ago I worked less and had more income. Something's wrong with the system. Everybody says it broke. In fact, I want to go on a four day week, take less money and enjoy life like I did twenty years ago. I don't want your dam resignation. We need bold guys like you."

The doctor kept his job. The meeting was a tipping point for the group. Leading is leading; managing is managing. Leading involves the future; managing involves the past, dealing with what is already established. The crisis led to a decision where every voice was heard and respected.

It is my contention that all physicians must become physician-executives, or physician-leaders. Healthcare in the hands of people who do not know the complexities of medicine is like asking a lipless person to play the trumpet. While there are those who disagree with me, I contend that every HMO, every healthcare system must be directed by persons with a medical background, even a medical degree, and every person sitting in the second chair must be experienced and degreed in economics and finance. The polarities of medicine and economics must be joined at the hip. They need not co-exist in the spirit of debate and dialectic. They must co-exist as the left arm does with the right.

Medicine and money will never go away.
"No margin, no mission" is a living reality.

Leaders must ask what is really going on, facilitating adept interventions and grounding their action in faith and hope. The issues of chaos, complexity, spirituality, evil, and theology must be addressed.

Leaders who have a deep sense of who they are and what they believe will be willing to listen to the stirrings of individuals and the organization. Leaders will know how to differentiate debate, dialogue and dialectic. Leaders will know how to make friends with polarity and paradox, to think inclusively and act congruently. Polarities can be managed. A paradox cannot.

Polarity and Paradox

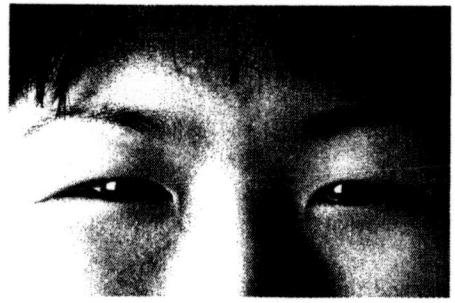

We have two eyes. When we see an object,
we experience one version, not two.
Two different eyes,
one version that produces depth
more powerful than either eye can give separately.
The power of paradox.

Chapter 10en

The Re-Birth Of HealthCare

Is re-birth possible? Can we agree on what it is? Do we need to engage in spiritual talk in order have a conversation about re-birth?

The notion of re-birth smacks of evangelists, large tents, altar calls, and public confessions. Aren't we too sophisticated for this? After all, we are an educated public and have the best standard of living in the world. So, why re-birth?

Let's begin with the **evangelists.** Remember the tobacco executives appearing before congress and were asked, "Do you believe that nicotine is addictive?" Every CEO answered, "No!" After these lies, we heard that "Project Whitecoat" was initiated by Philip Morris to orchestrate the controversy about passive smoking. As early as 1953 we learned about internal documents from the tobacco industry, which had knowledge of the detrimental effects of tobacco on our health. The headline was clear in 1953:

Industry acknowledges that smoking is linked to lung cancer

"... tobacco smoking is an important etiologic factor in the induction of primary cancer of the lung. Studies of clinical data tend to confirm the relationship between heavy and prolonged smoking and the incidence of lung cancer."

Claude Teague, Jr. February 2, 1953
Report to RJR Tobacco

The evangelists were from every segment of our society. They pounded the pulpit in earnest. "We're not going to listen to your lies any longer. We've had enough. We want you to confess, admit your wrong, so we can get on with the health of the nation."

They confessed. They lied. We knew they lied. They knew they lied. *And what did we learn?* We learned that the political process can and does work. We learned that some corporate leaders can and do lie through their stained teeth. We learned that the consequences for lying under oath have minimal personal impact. We

Re-Birth

learned that greed for money and position is still mighty powerful in the United States. We learned that the 'greater good' is but a paper value in the minds and behavior of the greedy.

We learned that re-birth of conscience is possible when confession is authentic. We learned that those without conscience can and will ruin the health of millions.

And what about **the tent**? The 'tent' used by the evangelist today can be a courtroom, a hearing room, a TV studio, a rally on the steps of the state house. The 'tent' is a gathering place for those with a passion to learn, a desire to commit, a yearning to make a difference.

The confession? Confession is an admission, an acknowledgement, and a declaration. The Greek work, 'hamartia' is the word for sin and it means 'missing the mark'. Our research reveals what many already know, namely, that we have missed the mark in dealing with:

- Learning disabilities in healthcare
- Losses of physicians
- Paradigm shifts

Healthcare has unraveled because it missed the mark. Somewhere, somehow, the patient got lost in the healthcare equation even though nearly every mission statement or corporate strategy declares that patient care comes first above everything.

Healthcare systems are not the problem. The problem is with us, consumers, practitioners, regulators. We can only point fingers at ourselves. To blame or single out individuals, departments, or institutions does little more than create additional derailments. Derailment is when people are excluded, history, even groups, are eliminated, where double standards are issued and supported, where oppression is practiced, where apathy is allowed center stage and where abdication of leadership is tolerated.

When we confess our derailments we address our dilemmas. When we address our dilemmas, we impress one another with determination and with determination we begin our journey. So, instead of

Elimination we have a shared history.

Instead of

Exclusion we have inclusion.

Instead of

Double standards we have justice.

Instead of

Oppression we have participation.

Instead of

Apathy we have love, concern, and compassion.

Instead of

Abdication we have responsibility.

Admittedly, this is the spiritual dimension of healthcare. Healthcare delivery, when focused on responsibility, compassion, participation, inclusion, and shared histories and values, will be reborn. The old will disappear in favor of something more lasting than the bottom line. To stand before one another, admit our participation in an unraveled system, be truthtellers, share our implicit and complicit involvement, past and present, in a less than perfect system, we can rejoice in a new beginning where the focus will be multicolored, and not just green.

Where do we begin?

We begin by determining what we have in common. What holds us together? What separates us? Is the question discussed regularly? What do we hold in common socially, naturally, and ethically? Garrett Hardin's article in Science (Issue 168: 143-148) talks about the *"Tragedy of the Commons,"* which links freedom with irresponsibility. Originally, "the commons" was an unfenced region of an agricultural community where everyone was free to graze livestock, raise crops, or gather wood; the upkeep was the responsibility of no one in particular and everyone in general. The "tragedy of the commons" is when self-interest takes land that belongs to everyone, overgrazes, clears the forest, before others do it. What is taken is not renewed and soon the commons are exhausted.

Hardin describes this tragedy as self-interest joining with mutual indifference. A commons area is developed either by greed or

Re-Birth

generosity, heedlessness or consideration, by self-concern or corporate caring.

Healthcare is currently in the grip of mutual indifference, greed, heedlessness and self-concern. We have all had a part in this. We cannot point fingers and get away with it.

Where do we begin?

By creating a "social commons," places that belong to everyone, where everyone is served, where everyone serves. Jedediah Purdy, in *"For Common Things"*, (Vintage, p. 99) calls this moral ecology. When we "act out of devotion to the common places, we act out of those things that enable us to trust and the bear the weight of others' trust."

We are 'free agents", free to be responsible and irresponsible. To be gripped by greed is to be free and irresponsible. To be compelled by generosity is to be free and responsible. Now, are we ready to begin together?

We begin by bringing together every conceivable stakeholder in healthcare. That's all of us! No one must be excluded. The table must be large enough for all of us, or those who represent us. This is too big for private industry. It is inappropriate for government to dictate the future without consultation. It would be catastrophic for individuals to assume responsibility for healthcare. It must involve all of us. All of us.

John F. Kennedy stood before the world and declared, "We will put a man on the moon and return him before the end of the next decade." He didn't have a clue as to how it would be done. He couldn't do it alone. And he didn't. We did it together.

We can also bring our history, our intelligence, our compassion, our values, and create the best healthcare system America has ever experienced. We can.

We can learn from the life and experience of physician leaders whose stories follow.

Chapter 11even
Physician Leaders

Throughout this book we've been talking professional and organization competencies. We've reviewed what it takes to be a robust organization and what kind of commitment is necessary to make a healthcare system worthy of being called great. I want you to meet two extraordinary people. I was fortunate to meet them through the Physician Leadership College at the University of St. Thomas and have the privilege of being in a learning environment where their intelligence, experience, and passion are evident in abundance. I suspect that you, too, can tell your stories of men and women in medicine who have made a difference to you and in your community.

Roger Gilbertson and Bill Peterson are physicians and physician leaders. Their lives and experiences are inspiring and instructive. Let me introduce you to them.

Bill Peterson is anything but ordinary. The first physician ever to serve on a public board of directors of a major community hospital, co-founder of a PPO, the first to start a quality assurance program at Abbot Northwestern Hospital, coordinated the long effort to develop the heart institute of Minneapolis, crisscrossed three states in order to develop business for the institute and provided leadership to purchase out state clinics which grew from solo practitioners to multiple staff. He was one of four from ANW in discussions that led to the formation of Life Span.

Unraveling and Re-Birth

In a serious effort to bring fiscal efficiency and responsibility to the purchasing effort, he worked closely with VHA (Voluntary Hospitals of America), an agency of several hundred hospitals working together for buying power and recruited a physician to head up the formation of a physician network to complement the hospital network.

That's an introduction to the life and work of a physician leader who began his formal work as a physician in 1945 upon graduation from the medical school at the University of Minnesota. His internship was during 1945-1946 at the U of M medical school. In 1946, he was assigned to the St. Cloud VA by army as a psychiatrist. His research was on the effect of ECT vs. insulin in paranoid schizophrenia. He founded the A/C Anon in St. Cloud and at the St. Cloud prison and discovered the potentially lethal effect of low potassium during recovery from insulin therapy. Following this experience he moved to a residency in Internal medicine at the U of M. In 1951 he was instructor and then assistant professor in charge of junior medical students in internal medicine. Bill was a founding member of Life Link, with Ramsey Hospital and the University of Minnesota. Life Link consists of fixed wing, helicopter, and ground ambulances.

As one of the founders of Allina, he retired in 1995, only to do more. He then assumed a half time job at VHA North Central and half time at Health Outcomes Institute (HOI) (Paul Elwood's understudy). He developed or helped develop standards of care, pathways, patient satisfaction surveys, outcomes assessment and disseminate them to partners and associates. He also traveled throughout Minnesota, and parts of Iowa and Wisconsin to form cooperatives among clinics; legislation enabled doctors to deal collectively as in buying or dealing with health plans. With H.O.I., he met with many clinics to apprise them of the patients' assessment of their care and met with them 6-8 months later to tell them what their corrective measures had accomplished.

He moved to the University Of St. Thomas in 1996 while maintaining an office at H.O.I., and VHA for several months Initially at University of St. Thomas, his responsibility was to maintain viability of short courses for the mini-MBA. He soon switched to an emphasis on TQM and CQI and then because of the long term frustration with the ineffective leadership with national physician organizations, he started what has become the Physician Leadership at the University of St. Thomas

He is a founding member of the Center for Cross Cultural Health, a founding member of the National Institute of health policy: University of St. Thomas and the University of Minnesota, on the original board of Park Place for Aids victims. He received the Shotwell award for contributions to medical care and a Consultant to BCBS for pathways and outcomes. So what drives this physician leader in so many critical areas of healthcare? It's constancy of purpose and the ability to get to what is really going on in, with, and between physicians and the organizations which both inhibit and support them.

Unraveling and Re-Birth

The values driving the life and activity of this remarkable physician leader are clear-cut:

1. What worked yesterday will be honored and likely ineffective today and certainly obsolete tomorrow.
2. Service is not optional.
3. Challenge the best practices and enhance them
4. Bring focus to everything
5. Open and fearless communication is the norm
6. Invent the future

Roger Gilbertson, quarterback and safety football star at the college-level is now an executive quarterback and safety in healthcare.

He has demonstrated his skills as a defensive and offensive team player who has learned that a group does not need a quarterback, a team does. Roger the quarterback has learned to read defenses and call offensive plays accordingly. As a defensive safety he is the one who protects the end zone against hostile opponents.

For 38 years, Roger Gilbertson has been a clinician, professor, executive, volunteer, family man and church man. As quarterback (CEO) for the largest hospital and largest medical operation in North Dakota and the largest hospital and multi-specialty between Minneapolis and the West Coast, the largest employer in North Dakota (4500), and the largest clinical teaching facility for the University of North Dakota school of medicine and health sciences, he knows how and when to listen to the coach (board), and to his teammates (staff), especially when the playing field is uneven and muddy, to the point of being unplayable.

Unraveling and Re-Birth

The sports metaphor is important for Gilbertson. While he has had considerable success in winning as an athlete, the critical learning for him is in the discipline and focus required to be a leader on both sides of the ball.

Gilbertson's values....
1. Honor the past without getting stuck in it
2. Build alliances with trustworthy people
3. Relationships first, all else second
4. Create safe places so risks can be taken
5. Listen, listen, listen, then speak
6. Teach and preach good news, use words if you must

The Author

Warren M. Hoffman, Sr. partner and principle of Zobius Leadership International is on the core faculty of the Physician Leadership College, University of St. Thomas (MN). He served on the core faculty of the University of Minnesota's School of Medicine program for medical directors for thirteen years. While an executive consultant with Personnel Decisions International, he conducted the research for this book. He remains with PDI's division of Career Management Services as an executive consultant.

He began his professional work as a United Presbyterian clergyman in Minnesota and Illinois and moved from the pastorate to the Executive Director of the North Central Career Development Center, St. Paul, MN, and then to the director of Leadership Development and Training for a Dayton Hudson operating company. His formal education began in Lennox, South Dakota, and then on to the University of Dubuque College and Seminary, the University of Edinburgh, Scotland.

He and Marian live in Shoreview, MN. They have four sons, and seven grandchildren. Marian, a professional musician (soprano), is graciously tolerant when her husband plays the piano (for his own amazement). Some say that he has a handsome twin brother.

Warren can be reached at warrenhoffman@attbi.com and www.zobius.net.

References/Bibliography

License to Steal: How Fraud Bleeds America's Healthcare system, Sparrow, Malcomb, Westview,
Severed Trust: Why American Medicine Hasn't Been Fixed. George D. Lundberg, Basic Books, 2000.
Managing The Medical Arms Race, Susan Bartlett Foote, University of California Press, 1992.
Deep Change: Discovering the Leader Within, Robert E. Quinn. Jossey-Bass, 1996.
Seven Zones For Leadership: Acting Authentically in Stability and Chaos, Robert Terry, Davies-Black, 2001.
Market-Driven Healthcare: Who Wins, Who Loses in the Transformation of America's Largest Service Industry? Perseus Pr. 1997.
Beyond Managed Care: How consumers and technology are changing the future of health care. Jossey-Bass, 2000.
Crossing the Quality Chasm: A new health system for the 21st Century. Institute of Medicine. National Academy Press. 2001
Evidence-Based Medicine: How to practice and teach EBM. David L Sackett and Sharon Straus, W. Scott Richardson, William Rosenberg, R. Brian Haynes. Wolfe Publishing LTD. 2nd Edition, 2000.
The Healthcare Value Chain: Producers, Purchasers, Providers. Lawton R. Burns. Jossey-Bass, 2002.
Managed Care: What it is and how it works. Wendy Knight. Aspen Publishers, 1998.
Oxymorons: The Myth of a U.S. Health Care System, J.D. Kleinke, Jossey-Bass, 2001.
Bleeding Edge: The business of health care in the new century. J.D. Kleinke, Aspen Publishers, 1998.
Health and **Health Care 2010. Institute for the Future. Jossey-Bass. 2000.**
Healthcare in the New Millennium: Vision, Values and Leadership, Ian Morrison. Jossey-Bass, 2000.

Global Health Care Markets: A Comprehensive Guide to Regions, Trends, Opportunities, Shaping the International Health Arena, Walter Wieners, Editor. John Wiley and Sons, 2001.
Polarity Management: Identifying and Managing Unsolvable Problems, Barry Johnson, Human Resource Development Press, 1997.
For Common Things, Purdy, Jedidiah, Knoph, 2000.